THE WISE SCALPEL

TIPS & TRAPS

in liver, gallbladder & pancreatic surgery

Francis R. Sutherland MD FRCSC

Chad G. Ball MD MSc FRCSC FACS

Illustrated by
Stephen P. Graepel MA

tfm Publishing Limited, Castle Hill Barns, Harley, Shrewsbury, SY5 6LX, UK
Tel: +44 (0)1952 510061; Fax: +44 (0)1952 510192
E-mail: info@tfmpublishing.com; Web site: www.tfmpublishing.com

Editing, design & typesetting: Nikki Bramhill BSc (Hons) Dip Law
Illustrations: Stephen P. Graepel MA
Cover photo: © iStock.com
Gallbladder human digestive system anatomy
Credit: myboxpra; stock illustration ID: 1267242950

First edition: © 2022
Paperback ISBN: 978-1-913755-12-6
E-book editions: © 2022
ePub ISBN: 978-1-913755-13-3
Mobi ISBN: 978-1-913755-14-0
Web pdf ISBN: 978-1-913755-15-7

Printed by Short Run Press Ltd., Bittern Road, Sowton Industrial Estate, Exeter, EX2 7LW, UK
Tel: 01392 211909; Fax: 01392 444134
E-mail: estimates@shortrunpress.co.uk; Web site: www.shortrunpress.co.uk

Contents

page

Introduction   1

SECTION I — HPB surgical craft

Chapter 1   Wisdom   7

Chapter 2   History of HPB surgery   13

Chapter 3   Multidisciplinary HPB teams   17

Chapter 4   Managing the operative environment   21

Chapter 5   Quality of HPB surgical care   27

Chapter 6   Operating with 'heuristics'   31

Chapter 7   Surgical skill development   41

Chapter 8   Technology: from electrocautery to robot   47

Chapter 9 Who should you operate on? 51

Chapter 10 Starting and finishing an operation 55

Chapter 11 The HPB 'complication radar' 59

Chapter 12 Giving bad news 65

SECTION II — Liver

Chapter 13 Liver anatomy 69

Chapter 14 Liver procedures 91

Chapter 15 Liver special circumstances 131

SECTION III — Porta hepatis

Chapter 16 Porta hepatis anatomy, procedures and 147
special circumstances

SECTION IV — Gallbladder

Chapter 17 Gallbladder anatomy 165

Chapter 18 The safe cholecystectomy (avoiding bile duct injuries) 171

Chapter 19 The difficult cholecystectomy 187

Chapter 20 Bile duct injury repair 191

Chapter 21 Gallbladder special circumstances 201

SECTION V — Pancreas

Chapter 22   Pancreatic anatomy   217

Chapter 23   Pancreatic procedures   223

Chapter 24   Pancreatic special circumstances   245

Chapter 25   Surgery for chronic pancreatitis   259

Chapter 26   Severe acute pancreatitis (riding the bull)   267

SECTION VI — HPB extras

Chapter 27   Other organs of the upper abdomen   281

Chapter 28   Dilated ducts and other oddities   293

Chapter 29   General surgery operations on cirrhotics   297

Chapter 30   The HPB surgeon in trauma   301

Chapter 31   Critical care and the HPB surgeon   307

Chapter 32   Pediatric HPB surgery   311

Epilogue   Parting thoughts   313

Index   315

Contributors

Authors

Dr. Francis R. Sutherland MD FRCSC is a Professor of Surgery at the University of Calgary. He has been a HPB and general surgeon for 30 years. He has broad experience training residents and fellows. He is a co-founder of the HPB Surgery Program for Southern Alberta and a co-founder of the Canadian HPB Association.

Dr. Chad G. Ball MD MSc FRCSC FACS is a Clinical Professor of Surgery at the University of Calgary. He has been an active HPB and trauma surgeon since 2005. He is the current Editor-in-Chief of the *Canadian Journal of Surgery* and Evidence-Based Reviews in Surgery Program.

Illustrator

Stephen P. Graepel MA is a graduate of the Johns Hopkins University School of Medicine, where he earned his Master of Arts in Medical and Biological Illustration. Mr. Graepel has worked as a medical Illustrator, art director, multimedia manager and a visual strategist, serving both providers and public health markets. He currently works with the Mayo Clinic as a senior medical illustrator with the Department of Neurosurgery.

Dedication

For my wife Linda — for her Incredible support, all the time.
Francis R. Sutherland

I would like to thank my partner, Dr. Francis Sutherland,
for his insight, generosity, and true mentorship.
It's been an amazing voyage together.
Chad G. Ball

The merit of all things lies in their difficulty.

Alexandre Dumas

Introduction

*The wisdom acquired with the passage of time
is a useless gift unless you share it.*
Esther Williams

OK boomer
Chlöe Swarbrick

Diseases of the foregut have always dealt man a challenging hand. Effective treatment for cancers, stones and inflammation within the liver, gallbladder, and pancreas have been slow to develop. For *Homo sapiens*, these maladies were historically a lethal event. The turn of the 19th century, however, brought real advances as surgery for many conditions offered improvements and true hope. Unfortunately, progress within liver and pancreas surgery lagged far behind. These organs, then and now, remain operative challenges. They are located deep within the abdomen and therefore discourage exposure. Both the liver and pancreas are soft and friable; not particularly good at 'taking a stitch'. Their anatomy is complicated. The rich blood supply, in and around their parenchyma, is daunting and there is no mesentery that allows the organs to be quickly mobilized and controlled. Finally, the liver and pancreas both have ductal systems that, once breached, have a predilection to leak substances of variable toxicity, including infected bile and pancreatic fluid. As a result, it has only been in the past 50 years that meaningful surgical progress has occurred.

➤ Wisdom

The liver and pancreas are not particularly good at 'taking a stitch'.

Significant progress in both anatomic understanding and quality of surgery has occurred via specialization specific to the liver and pancreas. Early on, a small number of operations on these organs were performed, mostly on a part-time basis by general surgeons. The evolution into a true subspecialty within general surgery occurred in some centres by design. However, in most hospitals, a more natural evolution took place. The reason for this progress is clear; the results of surgeons, not experienced in this area, were and remain poor. Large database studies in the late 20th century codified a clear volume-outcome relationship. The evolution of hepatopancreatobiliary (HPB) surgery has therefore moved through a number of steps. Initially, all general surgeons performed a limited repertoire of HPB operations, starting with cholecystectomy. This was followed by a 'go to' general surgeon, in isolated institutions, who concentrated more specifically on liver or pancreas resections. Eventually, that person was replaced by a surgeon who had received specific training in HPB procedures. Now, we see the development of teams of HPB surgeons working together with medical and radiology specialists, who have also obtained HPB focused training. Further evolution has centralized much of this care within a specific geographic region. The quality of surgery (operative outcomes) in these centres is now additionally scrutinized with the establishment of universal standards and benchmarks (NSQIP).

➤ Wisdom

HPB surgery has advanced by the concentration of care and development of teams.

The learning curve to become a HPB surgeon is steep. The hazards involved in these operations can be a painful experience with both real and potential (i.e., 'near miss') patient harm. This book aims to bootstrap learners in the basics of HPB surgery. It is not a textbook and it is not a 'how to' technical atlas, but rather a set of guiding principles, for approaching, understanding, learning and performing HPB surgery. We also review attributes that a surgeon must have to be successful, including a personal philosophy that supports wisdom acquisition. It must be remembered, however, that no amount of literature can replace one-on-one work with a surgical mentor. The procedures must be learned by following the direction of a 'master' surgeon. The apprenticeship model is still the cornerstone of training, especially in HPB surgery.

➤ Wisdom

The learning curve of HPB surgery is steep and full of horrors.

There are several horizontal themes in this book. All HPB surgeons are students of anatomy, so we never stray too far from the knowledge of critical structures. Be aware that this is applied anatomy; anatomy that is relevant to important surgical moves and maneuvers. It is essential that the surgeon knows more than just the most common layout of organs, but rather a compendium of anatomic possibilities. There is no 'normal' anatomy, only anatomical variations. This book concentrates on practical tips of operating within each different area of HPB surgery. These tips always tilt towards the conservative. After all, how we fail is of added importance for surgeons because someone else pays for our failure (we do not go down with the ship). While some techniques are described, these should never be considered definitive as there are many other equally viable approaches.

Traps are areas of risk that may not be initially appreciated. They are nasty corners within the surgical world that need to be completely avoided. Bypassing the mistakes of our ancestors allows trainees to move up to an elevated pathway in the search for competence. Bad experiences, though effective, are the bitterest way of acquiring wisdom. Lastly, this book endeavors to help young surgeons understand what they are trying to achieve and to develop a template for ongoing knowledge acquisition. We discuss some of the other required skills to function effectively in an ever changing modern surgical and social environment.

This review stresses a common sense approach. The primer is meant for 'mere mortal' surgeons who wish to perform these operations safely, rather than the aggressive surgeon intent on becoming a superstar, making their name by performing ever more risky procedures. It is important to remember that it is this bird that produces most of the chirping.

HPB surgery is about solving difficult challenges. Being a problem solver results in a life that is full of many arduous trials but brings with it a rich sense of accomplishment.

➢ Wisdom

HPB surgeons are problem solvers.

Wisdoms

- *The liver and pancreas are not particularly good at 'taking a stitch'.*

- *HPB surgery has advanced by the concentration of care and development of teams.*

- *The learning curve of HPB surgery is steep and full of horrors.*

- *HPB surgeons are problem solvers.*

Section I

HPB surgical craft

Understanding what we are trying to do is important. Before we dive into the details, we must establish a strong foundation of understanding and sense of direction. This will be the support structure for the details that follow.

Chapter 1

Wisdom

*Wisdom is not a product of schooling but a lifelong
attempt to acquire it.*
Albert Einstein

Wisdom seems to be in short supply these days. The process of acquiring wisdom does not even seem to be a remote goal as our world becomes more insular and technology driven. How can one acquire something as ethereal as wisdom? Indeed, why should we pursue wisdom at all? Perhaps artificial intelligence or the 'internet of things' will become the source of true wisdom. We may believe in this 'illogic' until we are facing a complicated operative environment, with significant uncertainty, and a stressed surgical team bordering on panic. Personal wisdom accumulation then becomes not just a thing; it becomes the only thing!

 Wisdom

Wisdom accumulation is the only thing!

What is wisdom and specifically what does it mean in HPB surgery? Wisdom is a way of behaving that balances multiple attributes that include basic and specific knowledge, common sense, insight, humility, and compassion. The traits of integrity and honesty are features of true wisdom. Wisdom is founded on reality and seeks to shed all the clutter of bias, ego and self-interest that affects our behavior. Wisdom allows one to make decisions on the basis of clear judgment and courage, the mental toughness to manage challenging situations and make difficult decisions. For a surgeon, wisdom requires effective self-knowledge and an ability to know what one is capable of. It seeks the best pathway for high-quality patient outcomes.

So how do we go about this long process of becoming 'wise'? Imitation is perhaps the easiest way to start this process. Spend time with someone who is wise and do what they do. Wisdom is 'foundational'. It has to have a very solid base upon which to add. Knowledge forms the base of the foundation and can only be acquired by dedicated hard work over many years. However, wisdom is more than just knowledge and requires a personal philosophy that molds experiences into our foundation. This philosophy involves taking personal responsibility for mistakes. Learning at every unfortunate turn fuels wisdom. Wisdom then becomes a set of principles that colors all of our actions. Wisdom in all its forms requires reflection, time spent sitting on a fence looking at the landscape of one's life and judging the direction of the winds of truth.

Wisdom

Wisdom in foundational.

The purpose of this review is to assist trainees in establishing this base so they can quickly start adding their experiences to a solid truth and a personal wisdom-based philosophy. It is a training 'heuristic' (more on that later); hopefully, a shortcut to real wisdom accumulation. The development of wisdom is not a given. Years of practice with 'non-seeing' eyes do not end in wisdom. Being self-critical and learning from our mistakes (humility) is the only true path.

➢ Wisdom

Wisdom involves knowledge and personal philosophy.

For a surgeon, wisdom is not just coordinated knowledge. It is a physical skill: the ability to dissect an area following a series of natural planes. It involves the capacity to navigate within a complicated three-dimensional environment, sense areas of hazard and avoid damaging the surrounding structures. It is a talent for taking things apart and putting them back together.

In our contemporary world of 'teams', wisdom is increasingly about interpersonal skill. Interacting with our colleagues and learners in an effective way will make the surgical care machine hum. Social skills pervade all aspects of our surgical care and can be as important in the outcome of surgery as operative skills. This is especially true in the palliative situation.

Possessing a model for acquiring and maintaining wisdom is useful. Of course, this is not an all or none concept. Some of us may be wise in some areas of our life and hopeless in others. The principles, however, remain the same. Wisdom starts with a series of individual 'experience blocks'. This may be reading, watching or doing something novel. They are not equal; clearly 'doing' is a bigger block than 'watching'. When we have a valuable learning experience, we must somehow incorporate it into our wisdom foundation. Our mind filters our experiences; some are retained and others are not. These 'filters' are attention and attitude. If we are oblivious to a valuable experience, potential wisdom just disappears. Hubris is like a lead shield; no experience blocks will get through. On the other hand, an open mind that seeks out new experiences will have more blocks and these blocks flow through more easily. Memory aids open our filters; keep a journal. We also are particularly prone to remembering stories. This is why reading around a case or reading to solve a patient problem has such impressive retention.

➢ Wisdom

Attention and attitude make wisdom happen.

Keep a journal and record your mistakes.

It is important to know that acquired wisdom is constantly being lost. Pearls are forgotten, skills degrade and knowledge becomes obsolete. Sometimes our attitude degrades into bitter disputes and conflict. Inordinate time pressures and burn-out kills wisdom. Wisdom requires a certain amount of introspection and self-care to keep our personal machines running in top order. Because wisdom blocks are constantly being dropped out, a process of maintenance is required. Staying even requires consistent lifelong learning. To continue to add to our overall volume of wisdom, however, requires significant effort. During early training, where new experiences are numerous, hubris is rare and the wisdom foundation is relatively empty; wisdom accumulation is rapid. Accumulation becomes more difficult as the number of experience blocks that are novel decrease. At some point, one must actively seek the 'novel'. Perhaps this even means reading a book on mindfulness or enrolling in a leadership course.

➢ Wisdom

Acquiring, maintaining and losing wisdom is a dynamic process.

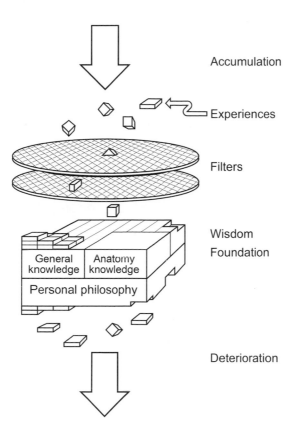

Accumulation

Experiences

Filters

Wisdom
Foundation

Deterioration

Wisdoms

- *Wisdom accumulation is the only thing!*

- *Wisdom in foundational.*

- *Wisdom involves knowledge and personal philosophy.*

- *Attention and attitude make wisdom happen.*

- *Keep a journal and record your mistakes.*

- *Acquiring, maintaining and losing wisdom is a dynamic process.*

Chapter 2

History of HPB surgery

You stood on the shoulders of geniuses...
Jurassic Park

The early pioneers of HPB surgery were largely surgical anatomists. Much of the original advances possess a distinctly French flavor, from Ton That Tung of French Indochina (Vietnam) to Claude Couinaud in Paris. Couinaud's book *Le Foie: Étude Anatomiques et Chirurgicales*, published in 1957, remains today the anatomic bible of liver surgery. The detailed diagrams based on 111 liver casts have never been equaled. Jean Louis Lortat-Jacob's first right hepatectomy and Jacques Hepp's bile duct reconstruction represent early surgical advances that were dominated by anatomic knowledge. In these early stages, cadaveric dissection and corrosion casts of the liver revealed the inner network of anatomy and underlying principles. Similarly, a knowledge of the underlying pancreatic anatomy allowed Kausch and others to perform the early pancreaticoduodenectomies.

 Wisdom

Early liver surgeons were all anatomists.

The early pioneers of HPB surgery possessed significant courage for embarking on a surgical cure for malignancies within the liver and pancreas. While gaining an understanding of the anatomy did allow for technical success, the lack of other support services that we now take for granted, often resulted in poor outcomes. Nutritional support, blood product administration and infection control were primitive in those early days. The development of pancreas head resection by W.O. Whipple could not move forward to a one-stage pancreaticoduodenectomy until the development of vitamin K therapy. In the early days of HPB surgery, significant complications had limited salvage options. Interventional radiology and critical care units did not exist. Relaparotomy was often the only avenue in a rescue attempt.

'Second-generation' HPB surgeons have added significant knowledge to move the subspecialty forward. These are the first surgeons to perform a high volume of HPB procedures. The relevant applied anatomy was defined and the steps of the procedures codified. Low CVP anesthesia was adopted and portal vein embolization was introduced. Names such as Belghiti and Bismuth are central. The Japanese married a detailed anatomic understanding with meticulous operative technique; Makuuchi and Nimura come to mind. High-volume pancreas surgeons (John Cameron) showed that it is possible to do Whipple procedures with minimal mortality. Because HPB surgery is largely practiced in academic centres, clinical studies abound. Many randomized controlled trials, initiated in this era, made HPB surgery more evidence-based.

The revolution of laparoscopic surgery is now well ensconced in HPB procedures. The pioneers showed real courage and a dogged persistence to push forward with the minimally invasive approach. Surgeons like Daniel Cherqui of France, Nick O'Rourke of Australia and others have pushed the limits of liver surgery. Michael Kendrick of the USA has shown the way, perfecting laparoscopic Whipple procedures.

This evolution of surgical skill in liver and pancreatic operations required several decades. Individual surgeons learned the bitter lessons of HPB surgery independently. Progress was steady, but painfully slow. It was not until the development of HPB training programs that more rapid advancement took place. Our new generation of trained HPB surgeons are now 'supercharged' as they put their foot down at the start of their surgical careers.

➤ Wisdom

New HPB surgeons are a product of evolution.

Technological advances have played their part. Computed tomography demonstrated the internal three-dimensional image of both the organ and pathology (cancer) with relationships to surrounding structures. This has allowed very careful advanced planning of surgery and not 'winging it' at laparotomy. It has allowed us to stay away from surgical misadventures in dealing with what often turned out to be unfixable problems. Energy devices have improved hemostasis; laparoscopy and robots have opened new fields of endeavour. Knowledge and technology now allow surgeons to push the limits of resection far beyond their earlier pioneers.

Wisdoms

- *Early liver surgeons were all anatomists.*

- *New HPB surgeons are a product of evolution.*

Chapter 3

Multidisciplinary HPB teams

*Remember teamwork begins by building trust. And the
only way to do that is to overcome our need for
invulnerability.*
Patrick Lencioni

The new reality for HPB surgeons is working within a team of specialists to provide care for a complicated and diverse set of patients with HPB problems. While malignancy is often the overriding theme, infection, stones, and other inflammatory conditions can be equally (and sometimes even more) challenging. Surgery remains the central aspect of much of this care, but, the modern HPB surgeon cannot be the stand-alone fiercely independent practitioner of the past. Modern high-quality care can only be delivered from within a group setting.

As a group, HPB patients tend to be elderly. Significant patient comorbidities, in a modern HPB practice, tend to be the rule rather than the exception. Formal preoperative assessment and risk stratification by our medical colleagues can bring the most 'tuned' patients into the operating theatre and help manage ongoing perioperative medical conditions. Our radiology partners perform numerous critical preoperative interventions such as biliary drain placement and/or portal vein embolization. Endoscopic ultrasound, biopsy and stent placement by our gastrointestinal colleagues also provide essential services. Neoadjuvant chemotherapy offers realistic hope for locally advanced pancreatic/liver tumors and prolongs life in the adjuvant setting in most HPB cancers. Experienced anesthesiologists can smooth a difficult operation, and our critical care colleagues can salvage patients in dire postoperative situations.

 ## Wisdom

What part of the word 'team' do you not understand?

The multidisciplinary HPB team is a team like no other. The members may not know each other well and spend most of their time working within their own specialty. The group is dynamic as members come and go with junior and senior learners (and even staff) participating on a rotational basis. There is no boss to manage the group and inevitable interpersonal conflicts. Historical hostilities and misunderstandings may permeate the present. There may be an underlying competition for patient referrals, within the group and even between surgeons. Participation within the group is often voluntary and can be withdrawn if an individual feels slighted. It is therefore important to be conscious of group dynamics and pay attention to the crucial conversations that are taking place.

Understanding group dynamics and how functional teams communicate is a skill that HPB surgeons must master. A non-threatening environment where team members can speak their opinions and voice concerns improves patient safety. It is important to insert your opinion into the pool carefully, strong enough to be heard but not too strong as to cut off other meaningful discussion.

Wisdom

Throw your opinion into the 'pool' with care; make the right amount of ripples.

Having constructive disagreements (conflict) is an important part of a functional team. The team must be able to work through difficult issues to come up with a patient plan that is acceptable. If members of the team do not feel safe to speak up, potential clinical mistakes may proceed to patient harm. Our quality of working life is largely dependent on our team dynamics. As with any neighbor, winning an argument or conflict is much less important than having good relations. Every team member should read the book *Crucial Conversations*.

➢ Wisdom

Constructive 'conflict' only; do not try to win an argument with team members.

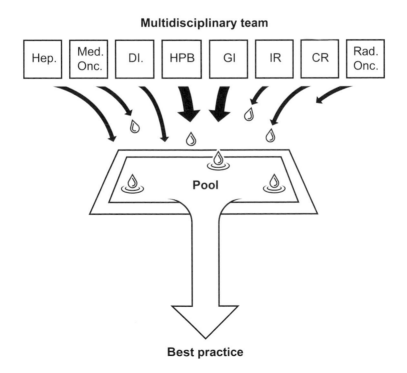

Wisdoms

- *What part of the word 'team' do you not understand?*

- *Throw your opinion into the 'pool' with care; make the right amount of ripples.*

- *Constructive 'conflict' only; do not try to win an argument with team members.*

Chapter 4

Managing the operative environment

Anyone can hold the helm when the sea is calm.
Publilius Syrus

Mindfulness has become popular in recent self-improvement literature. Being aware and 'in the moment' does have distinct advantages for a surgeon hoping to control their operative environment. A high degree of situational awareness allows a surgeon to fine-tune behavior that enhances team cohesiveness and function.

In the operating room, the surgeon still maintains some pre-eminence. Really, surgeons are the only person that can affect the end result. It is a mistake to consider the OR table like an airplane cockpit with interchangeable pilots. In the OR there is only one pilot and while assistants and residents can offer useful insights, they do not have the depth of knowledge to be considered 'co-pilots'. The only way to have a true co-pilot is to invite an HPB colleague to assist in difficult operations or situations of complicated decision making. Honest, real-time opinions from colleagues are part of a high-quality program. This only occurs when there is a safe, supportive comfort zone between staff surgeons.

➤ Wisdom

You are the pilot; there is no co-pilot.

A team is a group of individuals that work together to obtain a favorable outcome. A real team produces synergy: more than the sum of its parts. The operating room 'teams' are uniquely composed of small, malleable, ever-changing groups of individuals. Making a real team requires management with up-front conversations about the role of each member. Acknowledging and engaging every individual makes for a cohesive team. These crucial communications must take place prior to beginning an operation. In busy clinical services, these interactions are often neglected; on the ward regular short team meetings are also essential.

➤ Wisdom

An operating room 'group' requires leadership work to become a 'team'.

Team members will have different levels of expertise and competence. Respectful treatment of all team members is indispensable. Denigration or humiliation of lesser performers destroys the morale of the whole team. The top team members are often not the 'superstars'. The best rugby team in the world, the New Zealand All Blacks, does not always include the best players in the country. A patient first attitude and maximizing learning for each team member are key goals for the team and are not mutually exclusive. Engaging your nursing staff will mean that breaks will not be planned during critical parts of the operation. The scrub nurse can also have that vascular stitch 'loaded for action' and on the table.

➢ Wisdom

Leadership is about pre-emptive communication.

The Surgical Safety Checklist is as much a social event as it is a safety event. It is a great opportunity to show respect to everyone in the room in an effort to bring them onside and create a happy work environment. It is an opportunity to lead. Some things have to be said and not just implied. Learning names is like magic for team cohesiveness. This sets the stage for when there are real problems and the team needs to work together. In a critical situation, early, calm and rational communications with the OR team will improve the outcome. Do not forget that you are the leader and the team will take its cues from you.

➢ Wisdom

In an emergency situation, the surgeon's voice is a powerful tool.

Surgeons have been doing their own checklists long before the World Health Organization was involved. We review the history, preoperative consultations, and all diagnostic imaging. We check the consent (if there is anything during the work-up that you wish to remember always put it on the consent). Communicate your requirements to the OR staff and anesthesia early, long before the official Surgical Safety Checklist (maybe even the week before). You must reassure the patient face to face in the operating theatre. Mediocrity is not an option.

Wisdom

Do your own private pre-op checklist.

Checklists are not just about ticking boxes. The important issue is for the team to internalize the message of 'conscious scrutiny of what is going on'. It is easy to fall into a routine and stop seeing the room for what it is, from the little things that make the environment safe to an overall picture and level of efficiency. The reduced mortality documented with the implementation of the WHO Surgical Safety Checklist likely has nothing to do with each individual 'tick'. After all, a mandatory box will always be ticked as everyone knows it will be recorded as a quality indicator (tick box fraud). The safety culture is as much a personal commitment as it is a team conviction.

Interacting with technology is a necessary part of modern surgical life. Sometimes it turns ugly. Special tools, cameras and monitors, cautery, etc., all have a propensity to malfunction. Do not proceed until you are sure everything you need is present and working. If not, sit down and have a pleasant break while waiting for the items you need. Showing your displeasure does not move things along. Most surgeons, by necessity, have a trouble-shooting algorithm for misbehaving technology. HPB surgeons must have a deep understanding of the tools they employ.

Wisdom

Know your tools.

Wisdoms

- *You are the pilot; there is no co-pilot.*

- *An operating room 'group' requires leadership work to become a 'team'.*

- *Leadership is about pre-emptive communication.*

- *In an emergency situation, the surgeon's voice is a powerful tool.*

- *Do your own private pre-op checklist.*

- *Know your tools.*

Chapter 5

Quality of HPB surgical care

Quality means doing it right when no one is looking.
Henry Ford

A program that delivers clinical services starts and ends with high-quality patient care. Whenever a decision has to be made, a patient-centric thought process is what matters. This is true for both administrators and clinicians. If an initiative does not directly improve patient care, then it is probably not worth the effort. Programs must have regular meetings with safe and open conversations about clinical plans and pathways. This may seem intuitive, but on a busy and hectic service it is the easiest thing to neglect. Clinical staff can be overwhelmed with the volume and the high acuity of HPB patients and their problems.

 Wisdom

Communicate with your ever changing surgical team.

Regular review of unbiased outcome data with comparisons to evolving standards set by the HPB community are becoming more common. Each member of the surgical team must take ownership of the group results. Being invested in a colleague's patients fosters critical communication. In this way the outcome of each patient becomes the responsibility of all members of the team. Multiple eyes improve both individual and collective decision making.

 Wisdom

Take responsibility for 'team' results.

Knowing personal results, with comparison to colleague benchmarks, also breeds quality. Our former chief of surgery used to send out a yearly breakdown of each surgeon's wound infection rate with a comparison to the collective rates of colleagues. This was powerful behavior changing information. Sometimes we are not as great as we imagine in our own minds.

 Wisdom

Know your own results.

Communicating with patients and families is a central part of team activity. It must be led by the staff surgeon so that the messages are consistent. While much of the day-to-day information can be provided by residents and other students, key messaging should originate from the staff surgeon. Many HPB problems are not solvable; these patients must still receive the message of ongoing support and empathy. Giving this message should not be left to the most junior member of the team. When complications arise or things are simply not going well, communication has to go up the line of responsibility.

Wisdom

Critical communication moves uphill.

Quality improvement cannot be realized by large department-led initiatives alone. To be effective the process must be driven by small teams. Surgeons leading this voyage make it happen. Be a champion of change; encourage those changes that improve patient outcomes. Your attitude will be internalized by every member of the team.

 Wisdom

Be a champion of change.

Wisdoms

- *Communicate with your ever changing surgical team.*

- *Take responsibility for 'team' results.*

- *Know your own results.*

- *Critical communication moves uphill.*

- *Be a champion of change.*

Chapter 6

Operating with 'heuristics'

By their very nature, heuristic shortcuts will
produce biases...
Daniel Kahneman

Homo erectus, on the African savannah two million years ago, developed a style of behavior that maximized the chances of survival. This style is embedded within our genes. Man largely survived on the basis of his intellect: his ability to plan and to anticipate what comes next. This requires the storage of a large amount of information. Two things made this possible. Man developed a large brain with significant storage room. Even this large brain was not enough to store information about all possible situations, so a system of schematizing information evolved. Putting situations into similar groups allows application of a generic response. This created the capacity to retain a full and comprehensive mental library of different situations. Then, in critical encounters with significant ambiguity or limited information, rapid mental processing could complete the perception by making assumptions. This allowed an immediate physical response. An ambiguous percept was not compatible with survival so early man learned to take the probable and make it definite. The harsh reality of the environment did not afford our ancestors the opportunity to take a second look. Speed was safety.

Thus, we evolved a capacity to shortcut our behavior with very little conscious thought. We have a proficiency for automatic, intuitive responses. This allows us to move through our environment with speed. Cognitive psychologists have labeled these shortcuts 'heuristics' and surgeons live by them. Heuristics allow us to operate on minimal information and many assumptions. We are particularly good at seeing patterns where the signal to noise ratio is low and then move forward with authority. The efficiency of this system is impressive. While we are no longer dodging lions, we are now effectively avoiding 'tiger country'.

➤ Wisdom

Heuristics are an evolutionary gift to all surgeons from Homo erectus.

Cognitive heuristics

Heuristics can be divided into two basic categories: cognitive and motor. A surgeon's cognitive heuristics involves the use of stored imagery to navigate the operative field. These 'cognitive maps' are man's way of schematizing and storing the vast amounts of surgical environmental information necessary to operate. The maps allow the surgeon to quickly perceive structural landmarks. Superimposing a stored map on the area of the operation allows surgeons to make quick and largely subconscious assumptions about the anatomy-based limited clues. This makes the operation flow. Cognitive maps are the mechanism of our operative heuristics. Careful dissection and analysis of each structure would make for a painfully slow and arduous process; we would all be going home late. The 'intuition' supplied by these maps allows speed of activity. This works wonderfully, until it doesn't. It's not a foolproof system as assumptions and speed can generate mistakes. Cognitive biases make them worse.

➤ Wisdom

Cognitive maps are the mechanism of our operative heuristics.

While most of our cognitive processes are based on our visual perception of the operative field, haptics also play a role. The tips of our fingers contain a large number of sensory neurons. An expert learns to feel the tissues and planes that will separate or not. Palpation of the liver will deliver an enormous amount of information about how the liver will dissect and the position of the liver mass within the parenchyma. A slight indentation of tissue or pull will intuitively tell the surgeon how much tension to apply. Despite the 'no-hands' of laparoscopic surgery, haptics still play a part as the dissecting instrument is still connected to the surgeon's hand and some feel can be transmitted.

Cognitive biases are systematic errors that we all suffer. In certain circumstances we tend to make the same errors repeatedly and most of the time we do not consciously realize our defective thought process. Over two hundred such biases have been 'discovered'.

➤ Wisdom

Cognitive biases are 'systematic' errors we all make.

Four of the cognitive biases that are important for surgeons are primacy, availability, action, and confirmation. Primacy is the bias that what we see first has an overwhelming effect on our subsequent interpretations. We tend to get stuck on our first impression and then have difficulty changing our minds. We have a very strong capacity to believe what we see; disbelieving requires hard effortful thought. Availability bias emphasizes our inability to construct alternative scenarios or plans of action after starting down a path. Other possibilities do not come to mind as our attention becomes narrow. Action is a bias that is strongly represented in surgical psyche. The urge to just 'do something' may overwhelm thoughtful contemplation of a problem. Surgery probably selects individuals with a propensity for this bias. Lastly, confirmation bias is our ability to interpret all new information to support our chosen path, despite evidence to the contrary. It is this cognitive fixation and plan continuation that is responsible for many of our gravest errors.

 ## Wisdom

Confirmation bias is the interpretation of all future information to confirm a preconceived assumption.

The only strategy for surgeons to avoid our ancestry of heuristics and bias is to take a time-out. You will no longer be eaten when you pause to take a second look. A time-out can vary from a slow down to a complete stop. It may even require obtaining another set of experienced eyes on the problem. Time-outs are essentially debiasing strategies that take us from fast automatic heuristic thought to slow analytical and effortful thinking. Daniel Kahneman labeled these type I (fast) and type II (slow) thinking, respectively. In a difficult spot, experienced surgeons slow and focus all their attention on the task. At other times, perhaps at a critical juncture in the operation, we have to regiment ourselves to stop and review the situation before proceeding.

A surgeon's attention capacity is fixed. We can only think about so much at one time and when our attention bucket is full, critical information may flow out of the bucket. We get more and more focused on one thing. This tunnel vision occurs as we blank out surrounding aspects of our work. Important aspects of our operation are out of mind as we focus on a deep bleeding vessel. Fortunately, our bucket is usually only partly full as we do the more routine parts of the operation on 'automatic'. This leaves essential room for expanding our thinking in critical times. A trainee who has their attention bucket full most of the time does not have this capacity.

This new understanding of our cognitive processes gives us some insight into how complications occur. As we move along in our operation, rapid moves result in minor mistakes. These mistakes happen because heuristics are imperfect. A short 'slow down' usually allows quick correction. A dissection plane is rediscovered or a small blood vessel is cauterized. This process of repeated 'mini time-outs' and correction are occurring all the time. At some point, perhaps, a mistake occurs that is not corrected. No time-out occurs, and the operation proceeds down the wrong path. It is here that our innate cognitive biases may prevent correction. We interpret new information to conform with our misinterpretation of reality, we do not see the alternatives and we push forward with our fixed interpretation. Further on, more mistakes and lack of correction eventually do patient harm. The other possibility is that we have allowed our heuristics to develop into a bad habit, a shortcut that is dangerous. This results in a big mistake that causes immediate harm.

To avoid complications, some overriding speed control is necessary to reduce the number of mistakes and allow for mini time-outs to occur. A full stop safety time-out must be incorporated into the critical moments of all operations. Cognitive bias control is an ongoing process of time-outs with both slow downs and stops. Bad habits are particularly difficult to exterminate. Perhaps a regular review of our operating room skills and coaching by colleagues is an idea whose time has come.

➤ Wisdom

Take a time-out to control your own raging 'cognitive biases'.

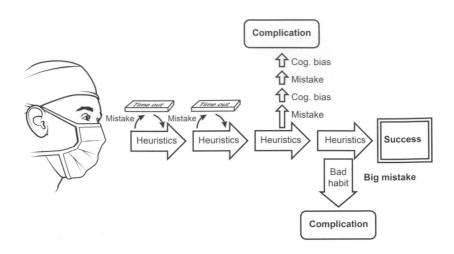

Motor heuristics

Motor heuristics are what surgeons do intuitively with their body movement, from posture to fine finger motor movements. Like all heuristics, it is subconscious, so surgeons cannot tell you what they are doing. Posture is perhaps the most unstated heuristic. Generally, master surgeons stand erect with their arms at their side. You cannot bend over for a four-hour operation and expect your back to remain functional. Resting arms at the side of the body provides support and better control. Elbows out (winging) will create neck and shoulder problems. The least distance between the action (i.e., cautery tip) and the supported structure (fulcrum), the more control there is. The longer this distance, the more our inherent tremor is amplified and control is reduced. Resting a hand or forearm on the patient reduces tremor and enhances control. Similarly, placing the needle driver closer to the needle tip increases control.

> ## Wisdom

The shortest fulcrum means the most control.

The table position and lighting are much neglected heuristics. The table must be at a height that allows elbows to remain at the surgeon's side and a forearm resting place to reduce fulcrum distance. Operating lights for most HPB operations need to angle the light upwards into the subcostal darkness.

A surgeon's position will change depending on what they are trying to accomplish. Shifting feet and body position allows the lever arm to be placed in the most advantageous ergonomic position. Moving or tipping the patient or even standing on a stool are all part of surgical ergonomics. If the patient can't be moved, often their organs can be placed in the best position with retractors or packs.

➤ Wisdom

Surgeon body position is an important motor heuristic.

The actual HPB operation with the separation of tissues is dominated by the fact that these organs are fixed in the retroperitoneum. Traction is necessary to divide tissues along planes of least resistance. Learning how much traction or pressure to apply is difficult as differences are often supple and unappreciated until the tissues tear. Because of the fixed nature of liver and pancreas organs, simply pulling the tissues in one direction with a hand or instrument will suffice to create a tension plane. The tissues are then divided at right angles to these tension lines. This can be done with a knife or scissors; most HPB surgeons have developed their skills with unipolar electrocautery (diathermy) to do this. The application of low alternating current to tensioned tissues vaporizes one thin layer of tissue at a time without causing damage to underlying structures. There is no 'char' created.

Sometimes blunt dissection with a 'peanut' or tip of a right angle can be necessary around critical vascular structures. HPB surgeons often use the 'spatula' of the cautery to perform a rapid combination of blunt and diathermy dissection. The right angle is now largely used only to encircle structures.

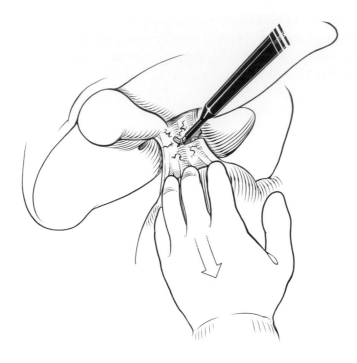

➤ Wisdom

Tissues are divided at right angles to lines of tension.

As one works their way through tissues, inevitable blood vessels present. These can be controlled with cautery, clips, ties or sutures. The intuitive knowledge of when to use each takes time to internalize. Pre-emptive suturing or tying a critical vessel prior to dissection is a hallmark of wisdom. The simple placement of a clip requires skill. The structure to be clipped must not move! Torquing causes bleeding. Pinch burning, a staple of general surgery, is less useful in HPB surgery as it creates too much collateral burn (heat sync) to critical structures.

Suturing liver and pancreas requires special skill and patience. Sutures must be placed exactly and removed from the tissue 'on the curve'. Any tearing will result in leakage of horrible things. The tension needed for tying anastomotic sutures must be exact.

➢ Wisdom

The HPB needle always exits 'on the curve'.

The application of stapling devices is a huge and conscious time saver. However, some tissues staple well and some do not. Staplers will fail if used incorrectly. A clip placed around the area to be stapled is perhaps the most common cause of failure as it prevents proper staple closure. Slipping a stapler into a defined hole to control bleeding requires heuristic finesse.

Laparoscopic procedures change the motor heuristics of operating. The critical use of gravity by patient positioning allows some exposure in the absence of fixed retractors. Laparoscopically, it is more difficult to create a tension line so the use of a sealing device is more common. This is also important as bleeders are more difficult to control. The magnification and lighting from the camera creates different shadows and a different image than an open procedure. These changes must be incorporated in the retained imagery used in the surgeon's cognitive map. The reduction of haptics (feeling the tissues) makes these procedures largely visual. The nature of tissues cannot be easily felt so a technique to indent the tissue with the instrument must be learned. Intraoperative ultrasound must replace bimanual palpation. By their very nature laparoscopic procedures increase the length of the fulcrum and increase hand tremor making basic moves and suturing more difficult. The long fulcrum arm of laparoscopic instruments also significantly increases pressure on the effector tip of the instrument. This explains why learners often initially pull too hard on critical structures. To a certain extent, robots fix these problems.

➤ Wisdom

Open surgery cognitive maps must be adjusted to the laparoscopic environment.

Wisdoms

- *Heuristics are an evolutionary gift to all surgeons from Homo erectus.*

- *Cognitive maps are the mechanism of our operative heuristics.*

- *Cognitive biases are 'systematic' errors we all make.*

- *Confirmation bias is the interpretation of all future information to confirm a preconceived assumption.*

- *Take a time-out to control your own raging 'cognitive biases'.*

- *The shortest fulcrum means the most control.*

- *Surgeon body position is an important motor heuristic.*

- *Tissues are divided at right angles to lines of tension.*

- *The HPB needle always exits 'on the curve'.*

- *Open surgery cognitive maps must be adjusted to the laparoscopic environment.*

Chapter 7

Surgical skill development

The greatest carver does the least cutting.
Lao-Tzu

When one begins the process of learning HPB surgery, one might think there is a pathway that first arrives at competence and then moves forward to mastery. However, technical and cognitive skill development is an inexact science that must be individualized for each learner. We all have different inherent ways of learning and start at different levels of ability. We run at different speeds along different paths and only at the finish line, a completed operation, are things the same. There is no 'one way' to successfully complete an operation, but there are certainly logical and efficient steps that all master surgeons hold in common. Poor and less efficient pathways are available for the lazy learner.

Probably the most important thing for an HPB surgical trainee is to gain a superb understanding of the immediate environment within which they must operate. All trainees must become students of anatomy. This begins with book knowledge of named structures and anatomic variability. It then moves on to a more complex three-dimensional understanding of structures and their relationship to each other. Finally, it matures into an understanding of how the tissues behave, how they separate (or don't) and the hazards present at each location. Management of small problems so they do not escalate into large problems has to be experienced. These last levels of learning can only be developed by hands-on exploration of the environment. Simulation is useful for basic skill development but does not yet have the fidelity to accomplish the most sophisticated skill acquisition required for senior learners.

 Wisdom

Explore your HPB environment as often as possible.

You must do to learn; make mistakes and repair those mistakes. It is here that learning HPB surgery is difficult for both the learner and the teacher. Many of the anatomic liver and pancreas areas are unforgiving; mistakes can be difficult to repair and occasionally impossible. There are real patient consequences to making a hole in the portal vein or making a poor connection to the pancreas stump. Some parts of the operation simply cannot be redone. This makes the relationship between student and staff a key component of any training program. Trust and communication are essential. Allowing fixable mistakes to happen while avoiding the non-fixable is a challenge for every surgical preceptor.

➤ **Wisdom**

Mistakes are an essential part of learning.

Surgery is a wonderful environment for developing real skill and expertise. It is regular and predictable. Because most operations are repeated frequently, it offers the opportunity for repeated practice. Surgery also gives quick and decisive feedback to even the most inattentive learner. This feedback comes directly from the operative field (a whoosh of blood). Verbal feedback on a trainee's surgical performance is most effective when it is rendered respectfully by a trusted mentor. The earlier and more specific the feedback, the better. When we have a solid knowledge foundation, the addition of 'experience blocks' fills in and cements the edges. Each anatomic area becomes rich in meaning as more and more blocks are added.

When a student starts watching and then doing HPB operations, they are building up a bank of information that allows them to move within the operative space. As navigation is a central part of this process so is the development of cognitive maps. Storing these maps for future reference is the most likely mechanism. Cognitive maps are a stored representation of our environment. Consistent exposure and hands-on exploration allow our minds to develop these maps. It cannot be learned from a book or by simple observation. Nor can it be learned by undirected exploration. Hands-on mentoring with direction and meaningful feedback make it happen. Students that are particularly adept and learn quickly will gain trust and be given more exploration opportunities, while the student who requires more time will have those opportunities taken away. Careful monitoring of trainee progress is critical. There can be a tipping point where progress and gaining skill can tip into a loss of confidence and stagnation.

Wisdom

Build your HPB 'cognitive map' library.

When students start to learn this complicated surgery, it requires their complete 'bucket' of attention. Every move requires conscious thought. The moves are not certain and are often repeated with inaccuracies outweighing useful actions. Mistakes are frequent. It is a slow and painful process for both student and teacher. The goal is to develop familiarity and comfort with the areas of dissection and then with much practice, economy of motion; each move deliberate and effective.

Wisdom

The goal is 'economy of motion', not speed.

As we move towards efficiency, the process becomes more 'automatic' as deliberate thought is no longer necessary for most moves. We learn how much pressure to apply to effect the desired result. Our attention bucket is no longer always full. Patience and perseverance are necessary as this process is slow. Eventually we internalize an innate sense of how the tissues separate, connect and where the hazards are. This allows the surgeon to go fast in safe areas and slow down with more analytic thinking in difficult spots. Mistakes may still occur but they are recognized and fixed quickly. The use of landmarks becomes ingrained with each and every cognitive map that the learner stores. Perhaps after many years of practice the surgeon develops 'pace' so that the operation moves forward rapidly. A surgeon may even get to the point where they have 'flow', where the operation unfolds with very little directed thought.

A young surgeon or trainee may ask how they get through to the point of becoming a master surgeon and there is no easy answer. One must learn broad exposure, dissection planes, and when to use blunt versus sharp dissection. Electrocautery has become a mainstay of HPB surgery and must be absolutely mastered. Clearly, this requires a lot or work with seeing and doing hundreds, if not thousands, of operations in multiple different situations. But perhaps the key is to have the right learning attitude. This means being an opportunist to learn.

Wisdom

Be an 'opportunistic' learner.

If one is able to shed their ego and see the next patient or operation as the opportunity to learn, rapid movement along the ladder from novice to master will occur. Watching is only useful if the watcher's attitude is to be imminently prepared to take over the operation. Staff surgeons are less interested in a student's opinions of various techniques and more interested in their ability to listen, watch, learn and then eventually do. A hunger to see and do everything does not come across as 'brown-nosing'. A resident or fellow who considers they have found the answers, at any stage of training, truncates further development and discourages teaching. Attitude is everything; hubris is nothing.

 Wisdom

Shed your ego.

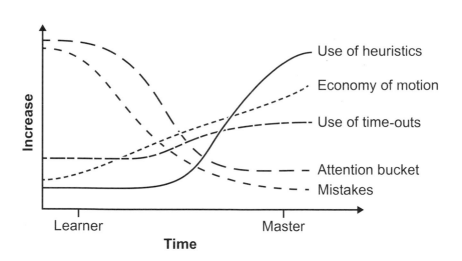

Wisdoms

- *Explore your HPB environment as often as possible.*

- *Mistakes are an essential part of learning.*

- *Build your HPB 'cognitive map' library.*

- *The goal is 'economy of motion', not speed.*

- *Be an 'opportunistic' learner.*

- *Shed your ego.*

Chapter 8

Technology: from electrocautery to robot

*If we continue to develop our technology without wisdom
or prudence, our servant may prove to be our executioner.*
Omar Bradley

Technology and HPB surgery are joined at the hip. Advances in HPB surgery are often tech-related. Electrocautery is one of those technology devices that HPB surgeons know intimately. The application of an alternating electrical current to tissues creates very localized heat and cell destruction. It can be used in several different forms: cutting, coagulation and fulguration, bipolar or unipolar. HPB surgeons generally use this device on a low current coagulation setting to divide planes and control small vessel bleeding. If the tissue is under perpendicular tension, this current allows it to separate with little collateral damage. HPB surgeons also use cautery at higher current levels to desiccate tissue and create a 'plug' for control of larger vessel bleeding. Unipolar electrocautery does most of the work. Laparoscopic liver surgeons have had much success with bipolar electrocautery to control bleeding. Learning the intricacies of electrocautery instruments takes years and a master surgeon often does this without thinking and so has difficulty conveying this knowledge.

Simple metal clips are a technology taken for granted. Rapid control of very small to very large vessels is possible. The art of clip placement (seating the clip properly and avoiding torque on the vessel) is rarely taught. Other devices have grown from the electrocautery base, including the Cavitron®, LigaSure™, Harmonic® scalpel, and Aquamantys™ (wet electrocautery). Each of these devices has advantages and disadvantages that must be learned. Stapling devices have revolutionized large blood vessel control. Clamping and suturing large blood vessels used to take significant time with increased risk of bleeding if the clamp came off.

Diagnostic imaging is perhaps the one technology area that has most advanced HPB surgery. Having an accurate three-dimensional picture of the upper abdomen is a game changer. The central place of CT and MR imaging in the patient with an HPB problem goes almost unnoticed in today's world. The traditional history, physical and investigation algorithm is often supplanted by an initial review of the CT scan. The discovery of a non-resectable situation should quickly redirect the patient's care. Indeed, the historical work-up algorithm is necessary only after a resectable lesion is found. While other subspecialties may have been just reading radiologists' reports, HPB surgeons have developed critical skills interpreting CT and MR images. Critical information is often not presented in the black and white report. Accurate imaging and biliary or abscess drain placement has revolutionized postoperative care. Sadly, imaging that shows recurrent disease usually means the end of surgical care.

➤ Wisdom

CT or MR images are now the beginning and end of all HPB surgical care.

Laparoscopy has revolutionized much of our surgical approaches. The only HPB surgeons that will not be performing laparoscopic surgery are those who are going to retire soon. Furthermore, your own personal robot is coming; get ready. Perhaps the major reason for this move is the surgical wound. Infections, hernias, and pain from abdominal incisions are significant and often understated problems after all HPB surgeries. As we add preoperative and postoperative chemotherapy to our algorithms, this problem may increase. Leaving the abdominal wall intact after a large operation is a laudable goal.

After the abdominal wall, the advantages of laparoscopy are largely visual. Looking around corners and into deep holes will move surgeons towards laparoscopic techniques. Magnification does have its advantages. The technology of 5mm cameras has improved to the point where they can be used to move around small ports for improved vision. Learn the tricks and practice suture control of bleeding vessels. The surgical principles of laparoscopic surgery are exactly the same as open; the standards are exactly the same as any open procedure.

➢ Wisdom

The standards of laparoscopic surgery are the same as open.

Truly virtuoso laparoscopic surgeons can do right liver and Whipple resections. These are highly skilled and motivated individuals who have trained and then practiced their craft. Doing these procedures with a robot adds a sense of 'Flash Gordon' to our surgical field. This certainly may become the standard of care in the future. In the early nineties, laparoscopic cholecystectomy very rapidly revolutionized gallbladder surgery. This laparoscopic HPB surgery revolution is happening, but at a slower pace. The question is not can 'whiz surgeons' get good results, but rather can this occur with the rest of us 'run of the mill players'.

➢ Wisdom

Laparoscopic HPB surgery is here to stay; get into it.

Wisdoms

- *CT or MR images are now the beginning and end of all HPB surgical care.*

- *The standards of laparoscopic surgery are the same as open.*

- *Laparoscopic HPB surgery is here to stay; get into it.*

Chapter 9

Who should you operate on?

Give me the wisdom to know what must be done
and with courage to do it.
Unknown

The practice of aggressive surgery often declines with the age and experience of the surgeon. You must monitor your own level of surgical aggression. Too timid and you may be missing an opportunity to cure or palliate; too aggressive and you may prematurely kill your patient. It is here that colleagues can be of great help — get a second opinion, before or during surgery! Fatally injuring your patient on the operating table or early in the postoperative course is soul destroying for patient, family, and surgeon.

➤ Wisdom

Be in the middle ground on the timid to aggressive scale.

The patient in your office with a resectable cancer deserves your careful thought regarding operative risk. Preoperative assessment by internal medicine and anesthesia colleagues can give us useful numbers to quantify risk; however, it is a fool's game to ask them to decide who should receive an operation. That is your job. The ultimate decision is often made by assimilating the risks and a gut assessment of the patient. How they greet you and enter into discussion of their problem can display a great amount of information about how they will do. Crisp, clear and direct answers are signs of a sharp mind that will motivate the body through any recovery, regardless of patient age. A sense of the patient's frailty can be intoned from their appearance and movements. Always watch as the patient moves from chair to the examining table (exam table test). It is a very informative part of the physical examination. If they can't make it to the table or need to be helped you better think twice about offering them an HPB operation. It is amazing how quickly the patient and family realise it's a test with everyone pitching in.

 Wisdom

Watch the patient closely: they will tell you their operative risk (exam table test).

Patients with dementia can often hide their real level of cognition with socially appropriate mannerisms. Partners provide cover by answering most of the questions. On the surface these patients may appear normal but any degree of dementia will manifest itself postoperatively. They simply do not tolerate major HPB surgery. If you are not sure of a patient's level of cognitive function, phone their family physician or have them assessed by a geriatric specialist.

 Wisdom

Patients with dementia are unlikely to thank you for your HPB operation.

Setting expectations with patients and family is not just a nice exercise, it is critical communication. The chance of death, overall risk of complications and months of recovery need to be spelled out. Saying, "If things go badly you may end up in the ICU on a ventilator" can really focus attention on the risky nature of these operations. While some numbers may help understanding, snowing the patient and family with rates of all possible outcomes is rarely useful. Most patients do not really understand statistics. For elderly patients it is important to first understand their level of function and let it be known that postoperative life may not return to that level. Some patients may lose their independence. Operating on a patient with a very low level of function may demote them to the lowest level of function, under the grass.

➢ Wisdom

Set expectations: discuss ICU admission and postoperative reduction in daily function.

Be real and try to help people decide. Meaningful communication results in realistic expectations. At the end of your diatribe, it is useful to give your opinion. After all, you are a consultant, not a statistician. Despite your best efforts, patients and family may demand an ill-advised operation. This does not oblige you to move forward. If you sense hostility and really do not connect, get a second opinion. Your partners will understand this request. They will respect it and evaluate you as a measured, thoughtful and clever surgeon. Occasionally, you will have to offer the patient another surgeon. You will never regret this either.

Wisdoms

- *Be in the middle ground on the timid to aggressive scale.*

- *Watch the patient closely: they will tell you their operative risk (exam table test).*

- *Patients with dementia are unlikely to thank you for your HPB operation.*

- *Set expectations: discuss ICU admission and postoperative reduction in daily function.*

Chapter 10

Starting and finishing an operation

Don't only practice your art, but force your way into its secrets, for it and knowledge can raise men to the divine.
Ludwig van Beethoven

The first part of an operation is a time of information gathering. Once things are well exposed, exploration will reveal the local extent of disease. What has been seen on diagnostic imaging is updated by the findings at surgery. A complete laparotomy will search for disseminated disease. Nothing goes forward until a hand or scope has evaluated the pelvis and diaphragm.

The first several surgical moves gives the surgeon a sense of his operative environment. Is it hostile or friendly? Most surgeons do a subconscious 'tissue assessment': How robust are the patient's tissues? How do they handle and separate? How much pressure needs to be applied to move the tissues without tearing? Are they friable or delicate? This is useful in setting the pace and style of the operation. Sometimes we can forge ahead quickly and other times we need to commit ourselves to a plodding pace while dividing dense adhesions. A patient with fatty delicate tissues is going to require more care. Some patients are just 'oozy' so we have to dedicate ourselves to ongoing bleeding control.

➤ Wisdom

Your 'tissue assessment' sets the style and pace of your operation.

When you are starting down an operative path that carries risk and uncertainty, 'bail-out pathways' must be kept in mind. When a 'commitment point' is reached (i.e., dividing the pancreatic neck) a time-out is totally appropriate. You have to ask yourself about your path and your patient.

➤ Wisdom

Learn the 'bail-out pathways' and 'commitment points' of your operation.

Obesity is an unfortunate reality in our society and is an increasing curse for the modern HPB surgeon. A layer of fat changes the operation in deep and drastic ways. One must first see a structure before it can be dissected. A layer of adipose tissue makes it difficult to find landmarks and expose organs. Control of vascular structures and making connections are hard. Strength and ultimately exhaustion may be factors in these operations.

Planning an operation in an obese or morbidly obese patient may require some modifications. First, it is important to discuss with the patient and family that obesity caries an increased risk of complications and death. Be sure that the time allotment for the surgery is increased. Pressure of time will cause mistakes and all obese patients require more time. Make the right incision: big. Get the right fixed retractor; multiple large blades. Use gravity effectively; get the patient upright by positioning the bed. Be sure to have the right assistants; tiny people sometimes make challenging assistants. Two staff surgeons that alternate can also be a successful strategy. Lastly, we should recognize our limitations; some things are not meant to be.

 Wisdom

Obesity makes you clumsy.

Finishing an HPB operation should initiate a number of maneuvers that all start with a time-out. Review the operation performed and ask yourself if you have done all that you set out to do. Check the consent. If there is something extra planned it should be written there. Go over any connections and look for blood or bile leakage that may need control. While extensive pawing around should be avoided, a gentle look will do no harm. Place the organs where you want them and ask if they need a stitch (i.e., suspension of the liver or closure of the mesentery). Irrigate to remove debris and ask yourself if a drain is indicated. Drains should be placed and secured at skin level as a last step so they are not dislodged. A double check on the specimens sent is in order. Review the disposition of the patient (ward, step down unit or ICU). The patient's volume status with early resuscitation plans and a postoperative analgesic plan should be reviewed with the anesthesiologist.

Early communication with the patient's family is an essential part of closing your communication loop. Feedback to your students and acknowledgment of your team is a professional responsibility and sets you up for success in future operations.

 Wisdom

Time-out the end of all your HPB operations.

Wisdoms

- *Your 'tissue assessment' sets the style and pace of your operation.*

- *Learn the 'bail-out pathways' and 'commitment points' of your operation.*

- *Obesity makes you clumsy.*

- *Time-out the end of all your HPB operations.*

Chapter 11

The HPB 'complication radar'

If there is no struggle, there is no progress.
Frederick Douglass

The early phase of a complication occurs gradually and then down the road it blows up suddenly. In other words, the patient becomes slowly more ill in front of 'non-seeing eyes' (confirmation bias) and then crashes.

➤ **Wisdom**

Postoperative problems present, gradually and then suddenly.

The wise surgeon has a radar that can sift through mountains of data and focus on the parts of a patient's situation that 'blinks' loudly on their screen. Patients may simply fall off the nominal pace/pathway of their recovery. It may be as simple as an inability to tolerate liquids or food. Paying attention allows early pick-up and intervention in the form of antibiotics, drainage and hyperalimentation; perhaps avoiding the need for critical care down the road.

➤ Wisdom

Recovery has a pace; watch for the patient who falls 'off pace'.

If a postoperative HPB patient becomes very ill, first ask yourself — are they bleeding? If this is not the case, ask — are they leaking? If you have ruled out these two things, call the internist and go home to bed!

There is much 'heuristic' truth in this statement and amongst the myriad of things that can go wrong, bleeding and leaking constitute the most serious. Fortunately, we have a vast armamentarium to address postoperative problems. Our radiologic saviours place drains and embolize blood vessels. Broad-spectrum antibiotics control infections and when things really go bad our critical care colleagues salvage horrendously ill patients. Our role is to recognize when things are going off the rails and get help early.

Preventing postoperative bleeding starts with the initial incision. Bleeding control is an attitude that permeates the operation from start to finish. It has to be an obsession, as a constant trickle of blood turns into liters of blood loss after a long operation. Attention to critical areas such as the GDA and SMA tributaries with appropriate time-outs to find and control errant vessels are essential. Anything that can go wrong, will go wrong. At the end of each stage of the procedure, a 'bleeding time-out' offers a moment to search for uncontrolled vessels. Do not wait for the end, as these areas may then be inaccessible. Gently rubbing an area of dissection may cause a tenuously controlled vessel to bleed and allow definitive control. Dry at the end of the procedure cannot be overemphasized. Large surgical blood losses are associated with increased complications and reduced survival. Some of this is undoubtably related to the bleeding itself rather than just the extent of the operation.

➤ Wisdom

Bleeding control is a procedure long attitude.

End the operation — 'dry as a desert'.

Instability in the recovery room should push the 'are they bleeding?' question through the surgeon's brains. The public shame felt from taking the patient immediately back to the OR is minor compared to the consequences of letting them bleed. Your colleagues do not actually perceive this as negatively as you do yourself. Low fluid volume anesthesia and epidural analgesia can lull us into thinking this is the cause of all postoperative hypotension. If suitable resuscitation does not result in a turnaround, think bleeding, check the hemoglobin. Late bleeding can be a bit of a surprise, but pancreatic juice where it should not be can erode any number of arterial blood vessels. This is especially true in patients who have had pancreatic necrosis debrided. Blood in the drains is a 'herald event' and means an early CT angiogram and embolization if a pseudoaneurysm is found.

Anything that man puts together can come asunder. A leak from a pancreas connection or stump can initially produce very subtle changes. The patient may be slightly tachycardic, short of breath or confused. These changes should be considered intra-abdominal sepsis until proven otherwise. Subjecting a patient to the ionizing radiation of a CT scan is less harmful that sending them to the intensive care unit.

Reoperation should always be a consideration in a failing patient. Early reoperation is much easier than delayed, where inflammation causes loss of clear tissue planes. Widespread contamination is best cleaned out by the 'responsible surgeon'. This decision will never come easily and should never be second guessed.

Surgically stressing elderly bodies can bring out any number of medical problems from heart to prostate. A team of other specialists in the hospital community are your back-up.

➤ Wisdom

HPB surgery makes people look their age and then some.

These problems seem to have a propensity to occur in the small hours of the morning. The overnight house staff need to be tuned into recognizing a critical turn of events. It is up to daily surgical staff to tune them up prior to the night concert. Recognizing that the patient is critical on morning rounds is an educational failure.

➤ Wisdom

The 8:00 AM emergency HPB reoperation means the wrong person was asleep at 3:00 AM.

Following HPB surgery, a patient may develop varying degrees of ascites. Most of the time it is nothing and resolves spontaneously. However, if a patient is unwell, it raises the question as to what the fluid actually is. There are several adverse possibilities to consider: infected ascites, succus entericus from a bowel leak, bile, or pancreatic fluid. If in doubt check the serum for bilirubin and lipase as they will be elevated by resorption. Otherwise, do an ultrasound-guided aspiration of the fluid for the real diagnosis (cell count, culture, bilirubin, and lipase).

Gastric outlet obstruction is common after Whipple or palliative bypass procedures. The longer the obstruction, the longer it takes to recover after a 'mechanical fix'. Blockage and dilatation of the stomach interferes with stomach motility and the new connection does not behave like a normal pylorus. Indeed, all patients have this problem to some degree. Time generally cures this issue. It appears that there is progressive improvement for 6 months or even longer; after a year most patients can eat normally. In the interim, various prokinetics and dietary advice can help.

Wisdoms

- *Postoperative problems present, gradually and then suddenly.*

- *Recovery has a pace; watch for the patient who falls 'off pace'.*

- *Bleeding control is a procedure long attitude.*

- *End the operation — 'dry as a desert'.*

- *HPB surgery makes people look their age and then some.*

- *The 8:00 AM emergency HPB reoperation means the wrong person was asleep at 3:00 AM.*

Chapter 12

Giving bad news

Give compassion with your ears...
Anonymous

Despite our best and most sustained efforts, HPB patients die at an alarming rate. After all, this is mainly a struggle against premature death and, unfortunately, death often wins. One must be in control of one's own emotions and be able to express empathy for patients in truly harrowing circumstances. How a surgeon handles 'bad news' situations has a significant impact on patients' lives, especially when a surgical cure is not an option. The trip to see the surgeon is often the seminal event in the cancer journey.

Perhaps the best advice is to be real and give the patient your time. After words of comfort and expressions of compassion, sitting in silence has value. Listen patiently and wait for questions; don't get ahead of what the patient is ready to hear. Don't let the patient's family or friends push you ahead of what the patient is ready to hear. It cannot be done fast and it cannot be done by the book. Remember that each patient is different. Some demand a direct blunt approach, whereas others require some soft stick handling.

Relieving suffering is part of your mandate. The patient in front of you may be experiencing pain, nausea, dehydration and many other forms of disability on top of the psychological trauma. It is your responsibility to make sure they are on appropriate medications and receive the appropriate care.

What support you cannot provide yourself, must be arranged. Some patients need to be sorted out as inpatients; so, admit them.

Perhaps the most comforting thing the patient can hear is that you will stay 'on side' for the duration.

> **Wisdom**

When giving bad news, be real and give the patient your time.

Wisdoms

- *When giving bad news, be real and give the patient your time.*

Section II

Liver

The liver offers resistance to the surgeon at every turn. It resists being seen as it hides in the right upper quadrant under the costal margin. It does not display its critical structures deep in the parenchyma and resists bleeding control with a generous and complex dual blood supply. Its friable nature resists an effective stitch. This resistant armor can only be broken with detailed three-dimensional anatomic knowledge. The liver has two central fixed vascular inflow tracts roughly situated above each other (porta hepatis and inferior vena cava) and one outflow tract (hepatic vein IVC junction). Liver surgeons spend their lives rotating the liver around these three tracts looking for the most advantageous angle of attack.

Chapter 13

Liver anatomy

Simple can be harder than complex: you have to work hard to get your thinking clean to make it simple. But it's worth it in the end because once you get there, you can move mountains.
Steve Jobs

Liver cover and attachments

The liver parenchyma is encased in Glisson's capsule and in most areas, peritoneum. The capsule and peritoneum are not the same thing. The capsule is a very thin fibrous layer attached directly to the liver parenchyma. It can bleed quite vigorously when stripped. The capsule extends entirely around the liver including the bare area and gallbladder fossa where no peritoneum exists. Glisson's capsule fuses with hepatic vein walls on one end and the plate system under the liver on the other.

The liver's outer covering consists of peritoneum which folds down from the diaphragm and abdominal/chest wall to encapsulate the liver; this effectively suspends the liver in the subdiaphragmatic space. The most immediately obvious attachment is the falciform ligament that connects the left liver to the anterior abdominal wall. It is basically a fold of peritoneum that hold the ligamentum teres on its way to become the left portal vein in the umbilical fossa. There is a variable amount of fat in this ligament. The left triangular/coronary ligament is also a partly fused fold of peritoneum that holds segment 2 next to the diaphragm. It is a wonder that we continue to label these peritoneal folds as ligaments, which they are not (including the coronary ligament, triangular ligament, splenorenal ligament, etc.). On the right side there is a similar fold but it is incomplete and does not cover the 'bare area' of the liver posteriorly. The first milestone of any trainee is to take down these attachments without doing damage. The two most common 'damages' done are making a hole in the left hepatic vein while taking down the left triangular ligament or making a tear in the liver parenchyma while dissecting the right bare area. The diaphragm (with the phrenic veins) from which the liver is suspended, is also easily damaged by the 'learning hand'.

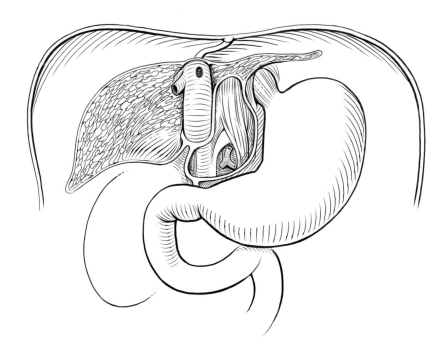

External liver orientation

Knowledge of the general layout of the liver is an important foundation on which to build anatomic understanding. The right liver is the largest and has an anterior to posterior orientation as it extends into the right subdiaphragmatic space. The left liver, with the stomach and spleen filling the left upper quadrant, tends to have a more right to left or horizonal orientation. It is thinner and more superficial and hence much more operable.

There are a few external clues to internal liver anatomy. Fissures are the major anatomic dividing planes between the different areas of the liver. The division of the portal vein is the most consistent compared to hepatic artery and bile ducts and is therefore used to label the major fissures. The gallbladder and space between the middle and right hepatic vein mark the main portal fissure. The origin of the right hepatic vein marks the right portal fissure. The falciform ligament and umbilical fissure demarcate the plane between segments 4 and 2/3. The posterior crease between segment 2/3 and the caudate lobe can be clearly seen with the ligamentum venosum deep in this groove. This is also where the lesser omentum originates.

Operating on the right liver requires that it be mobilised from its deep posterior location into the same horizontal plane as the left. The attachments to the diaphragm must be divided to allow the liver to rotate on the vena cava and porta hepatis. This rotation is only possible if the diaphragm attachments of the left liver (triangular ligaments) are first taken down. Mobilization changes the position of the right liver segments and hepatic veins relative to the preoperative imaging. With more extreme mobilization to visualize the vena cava, the posterior segments 6 and 7 become anterior. A lesion on the inferolateral side of the inferior vena cava (segment 7) is now above the vena cava!

The use of intraoperative ultrasound is important in reorienting after mobilization. Mobilization may also allow the surgeon to identify and orient the tumor. Finger tips are extremely effective tumor probes. With manual or bimanual palpation of a mobilized liver, surgeons can usually feel the tumor with their fingers.

➤ **Wisdom**

First get oriented and then get operating.

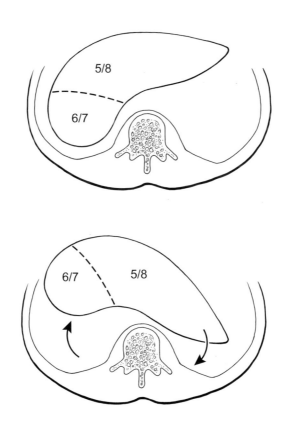

Internal liver orientation (obliquity)

A three-dimensional understanding of the internal liver is not possible without a word on 'obliquity'. The fissural planes of the liver, *in situ*, are not vertical. They are actually oblique in several directions. The main portal fissure, containing the middle hepatic vein, is at an angle from left to right. *In situ*, it is also tipped to the patient's right shoulder, off the coronal plane. The right portal fissure, containing the right hepatic vein, is almost horizonal *in situ*. The right and main portal fissures angle in towards the underlying caudate. This is intuitive when one realizes that none of the segments are square. In the right anterior sector, they are pie-shaped. They have a large surface area on the outside of the liver that narrows down as they close in on the vena cava. The shape of the other segments are all unique and unclassifiable in three dimensions. Even the hilum is oblique, tipped towards the right posterior subdiaphragmatic space.

When you divide the inflow tracts on either side of the liver, the demarcation line between segments and sectors is irregular. Rather than a clean plane, the fissural planes are an inexact wavy separation. The main portal fissure does not always end in the centre of the hilum (portal bifurcation). In about half of cases, it is either to the right or to the left. Surgeons should remember that the demarcation line (Cantlie's line) is just that, a line on the liver surface. It is a good start, but once one moves into the parenchyma plane, demarcation is indistinct and difficult to see. This is usually not a real problem as a moderate amount of devascularized liver tissue at the resection margins is well tolerated. Even larger areas of dead tissue do not seem to create a consistent issue; however, we should still strive to preserve only the vascularized tissue.

➢ Wisdom

The liver is separated by oblique irregular planes into odd-shaped segments.

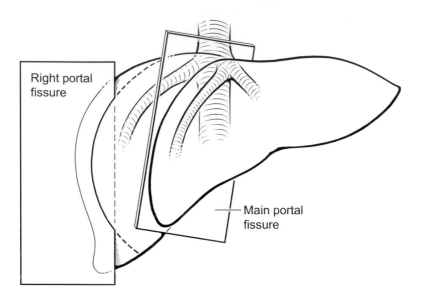

We operate on the liver in a number of different orientations depending on the amount of mobilization (i.e., movement and/or rotation of the liver). The liver goes up, down, left and right. This changes the direction of major hepatic veins and the dissection planes of the main fissures. For example, when doing a right hepatectomy, we mobilize the right liver, and make the main portal fissure almost vertical. However, when we perform a left hepatectomy through the same plane without right lobe mobilization, this plane remains oblique. Varying degrees of mobilization puts fissures and dissection planes at multiple different angles.

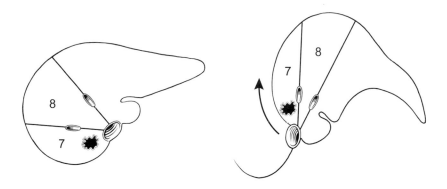

Humans are not particularly good with oblique orientation, irregular borders or odd-shaped segments. We have a bias to construct our cognitive maps in vertical and horizontal directions; angles tend to become 90°. In our minds we also tend to 'regularize' the images we interpret; we remember a cleaned up simplified version (squares) of what is real. Medical illustrators have the same problem, adding to the confusion.

Dealing with these cognitive biases requires significant work. Our mental representation of anatomy is often schematized; we have to spend the time to learn the real detailed anatomy and then transfer this knowledge onto what we are seeing at surgery. During dissection you may arrive at a major vascular structure you were not expecting; be humble and recognize you are lost. Take a time-out to reorient and get it right. Learn something new at each exploration, even if you are an aging boomer. Trainees must be given some extra time to work out this changing three-dimensional anatomy during exploration.

Plates and sheaths

The liver is unique for its paucity of surface landmarks. It is a black box inside that only becomes truly knowable as one works into it. The variability in position and branching pattern of Glissonian sheaths and hepatic veins are striking. There are, however, some principles that can help liver surgeons navigate this maze.

There are three structures that enter/leave the liver: the hepatic artery, portal vein and bile duct. They branch out in a variable tree-like pattern. This anatomy was discovered by corrosion casts of each tubular structure, separately. It was found that the portal vein has the most regular branching pattern so it was ultimately used to anatomically divide the liver into sectors and segments. According to convention we label the dividing planes between sectors: main portal fissure, right portal fissure and left portal fissure. The branching patterns of ducts and arteries are much more irregular. Because they were mostly studied in separate casts, the relationship of different duct, artery and portal vein branching patterns, under the plate, goes unmentioned. For instance, if there are duplications of the portal vein on the right is this associated with duplication of ducts and arteries?

Plates are thick fibrous shelves that form in critical areas where structures attach or enter the liver. They are separate from Glisson's capsule. There are four plates under the liver: the gallbladder plate separates the gallbladder from liver parenchyma; the hilar plate forms a thick demi cylinder above the porta hepatis; the umbilical plate is an extension of the hilar plate into the umbilical fossa and covers the vascular structures in the fossa; the plate of Arantius is simply an extension of the plate system from the umbilical fossa down the embryologic path of the ductus venosus to the left hepatic vein. It contains the ligamentum venosum. These plates are a short-cut to the soul of the liver and allow a surgeon to enter the liver in an elegant manner. All liver anatomic knowledge flows from the plate system and particularly the central hilar plate.

➢ Wisdom

The hilar plate is the entry point for key moves into the liver.

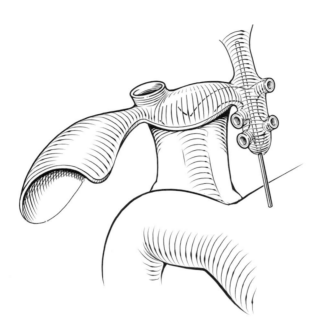

The structures of the porta (bile duct, hepatic artery and portal vein) push up against the hilar plate and enter the liver in right and left directions. On the right, they enter the liver directly, in a posterior direction. On the left, portal structures extend into the umbilical fossa and enter through either side of the umbilical plate. Small caudate sheaths enter through the back of the hilar plate. The area above the hilar plate (segment 4b) is largely empty of significant structures. No large Glissonian sheaths enter/leave the liver directly through the superior part of the hilar plate.

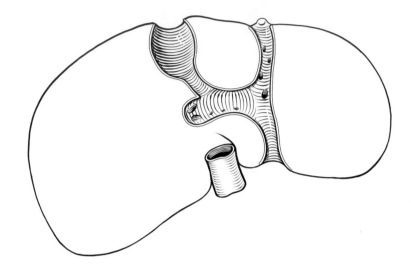

Of the three structures, it is only the bile duct that attaches itself to the hilar plate; it is difficult to separate from the plate surgically. Dividing the bile duct above the bifurcation requires division of the hilar plate. It is important to recognize that there is an impressive dense plexus of blood vessels within the hilar plate that supply the bile duct. Repair of bile duct injuries at the level of this vascularized plate is a significant key to success. This plexus of vessels is supplied by the right and left hepatic arteries; they form an important arterial bridge between right and left liver. When Claude Couinaud first entered the laboratory to study liver anatomy his first task was to study this vascular connection.

Within the liver, ducts and blood vessels do not occur by themselves but are wrapped together in a fibrous 'Glissonian' sheath. Conceptually, these sheaths form when the portal triad of duct, artery and vein takes the fibrous tissues of the hilar and umbilical plates with them as they extend into the liver parenchyma. Each of these 'vasculobiliary sheaths' has at least one portal vein, hepatic artery and bile duct collateral and supplies an anatomic area of the liver. Two or more hepatic arteries or ducts can be present in one proximal sheath. Above the plates, it is all sheaths and below the plates it is all individual vasculobiliary structures. Thus, anatomy tends to be extremely variable below the plate and much simpler above. There are no inflow vascular or bile duct collaterals between parenchymal areas supplied by Glissonian sheaths. Everything above a divided sheath is devascularized and dead. Johannes Walaeus actually first discovered these sheaths and some surgeons appropriately call them Walaean sheaths.

➤ Wisdom

Glissonian 'vasculobiliary' sheaths are the end units to each liver area.

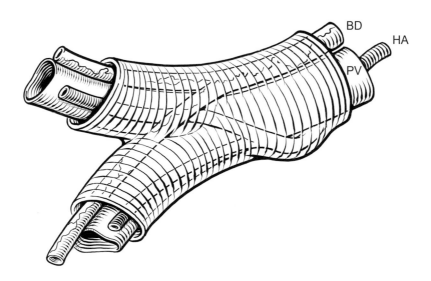

Sectoral/segmental anatomy

Anatomically, the liver can be sliced up a number of different ways. It is important that all members of the multidisciplinary liver team have the same vocabulary when communicating about the location of lesions within the parenchyma of the liver. The most anatomically consistent nomenclature is dividing the liver into three sectors: right posterior, right anterior and left. These large areas of liver are supplied by two proximal Glissonian sheaths on the right, and several umbilical fossa sheaths on the left. They are also separated by planes defined by the major hepatic veins. The right hepatic vein marks a plane of division between the right anterior and right posterior sectors (right portal fissure) and the middle hepatic vein marks the mid-plane of the liver (main portal fissure), the division between the right anterior sector and left liver.

Division of the left side is more indefinite, with the left portal fissure running between segments 2 and 3, along the tract of the left hepatic vein. The idea of a left portal fissure is usually ignored. Most surgeons appropriately divide the left liver by the plane of the umbilical fossa between segments 4 and 2/3. Thus, both inflow and outflow tracts are used to define the sectors of the liver.

➤ Wisdom

The three sectors of the liver are anatomically consistent.

In modern liver literature, sectors are often called sections. This creates some regularizing of nomenclature as it creates 4 sections. Hence a segment 2/3 resection becomes a left lateral sectionectomy, segment 4 a left medial sectionectomy, segment 5/8 a right medial sectionectomy and segment 6/7 a right lateral sectionectomy.

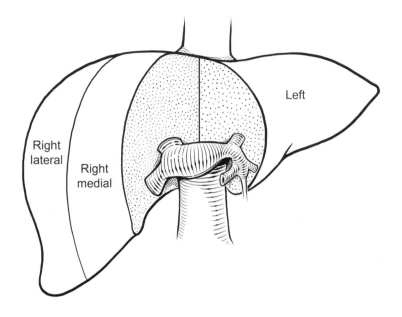

Segmental anatomy subdivides the 3 sectors. The hilum is the central part of the inflow vessels before major branching occurs. It is quite visible on all imaging and is a good landmark. The level of the hilum divides the right posterior sector into segments 6 and 7 and the right anterior sector into segments 5 and 8. On the left, segment 4 is located between the mid-plane (main portal fissure) and falciform ligament. Segments 2 and 3 are simply the superior and inferior part of the left lateral area. The umbilical fossa separates segment 4 from segments 2/3. Segment 4 is further divided into a superior 4a subsegment and an inferior 4b subsegment. The division between these two subsegments is somewhat arbitrary as there are no landmarks.

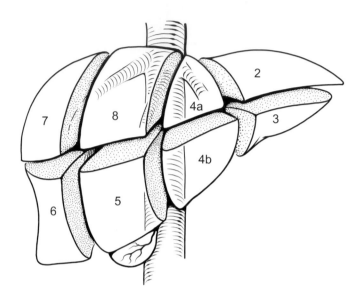

Controlling the Glissonian sheaths (above the plates) to sectors or segments is a useful technique. This must be done through parenchyma and is particularly facile in the left liver as the umbilical fossa allows easy exposure of single sheaths to each of segments 2 and 3. It is less feasible on the right where each segment has multiple sheaths originating from variable locations. The origin of these sheaths in the right liver are very deep in the parenchyma. Also, the size and shape of each segment on the right is extremely variable. Isolating the two larger sectoral sheaths on the right is perhaps more reasonable. The right anterior sheath appears similar to a mushroom giving off branches in all directions. The right posterior sheath is more like a Christmas tree with branches along a curving trunk. Once one has found the top of the hilar plate it is a simple matter of moving right to find the origin of these sectoral sheaths.

Glisson's capsule is the fibrous tunic covering of the liver. Stripping the capsule is for peritoneal surgeons, not HPB surgeons; it can bleed a lot.

➢ Wisdom

One sheath, one segment, is a myth.

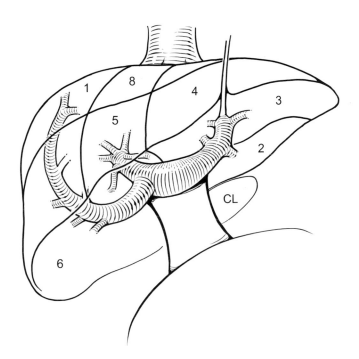

Umbilical fossa

The umbilical fossa has historically been labeled Rex's recessus. It can only be understood with a little knowledge of embryology. The venous system of the liver forms from both vitelline and umbilical veins that eventually fuse. In utero, a dominant umbilical vein develops to carry oxygenated placental blood past the liver into the heart (ductus venosum). The remnants of this structure form a straight line from umbilicus to IVC/left hepatic vein. It becomes the ligamentum teres, umbilical fossa portion of the left portal vein and then the ligamentum venosum (ligament-vein-ligament). It is a straight line.

The umbilical fossa gives direct access to the left liver. It is important to recognize that there is a single portal vein in this fossa that supplies both segment 4 and segments 2/3. If you wish to preserve any of these segments, this vein must be preserved with them. There is no such strategy as dissecting straight down the umbilical fossa; one always moves left or right to preserve this vein.

The umbilical plate is a demi cylinder that covers the structures in this fossa and is the barrier to entry into the parenchyma. When the left lobe is tipped up, direct access to the complicated interplay of vessels and ducts under the plate is possible. Getting on the parenchymal side of the plate simplifies anatomy and makes access to the segmental sheaths easy. It is possible to safely isolate and staple the entire inflow to the left liver at the entry to the umbilical fossa. Encircling the left side of the hilar plate extending from the edge of segment 4 and into the caudate allows the placement of a loop around all structures.

➤ Wisdom

The umbilical fossa is a rare anatomic gift to the centre of the left liver.

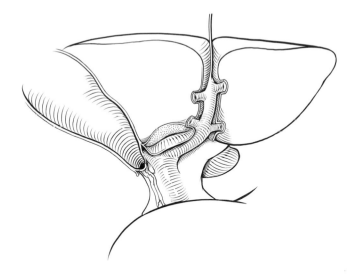

The caudate lobe

The caudate is a neverending classification nightmare. Is it on the left, or right? Is it a separate sector or a segment? What is its venous drainage pattern? It is perhaps an area of liver that stands on its own! Couinaud came to call it the 'dorsal liver' (previously segment 1).

Embryologically, the caudate forms by counterclockwise rotation of the liver under the inflow vessels (portal vein), outflow vessels (hepatic veins) and the ductus venosum. We should conceptualize the caudate in three parts, first, the paracaval portion behind segments 4 and 8, between the hepatic veins and vena cava. The second part is the Spiegel lobe which extends out over the left inferior vena cava. There is often an inferior notch between the paracaval and Spiegel areas. The third part is the caudate process which links the caudate to the right liver between the hilum and vena cava.

The borders of the caudate are indistinct. When dividing parenchyma there are no visible landmarks between segments 4, 7 and 8 and the caudate. The ventral border on segments 4 and 8 stays at the level of the ligamentum venosum. The right border with segment 7 is at the right side of the vena cava, and is also uncertain. The ducts and vessels that supply the caudate are numerous and arise directly out of both right and left sides of the proximal porta hepatis. They exit through the back edge of the hilar plate as small vasculobiliary sheaths.

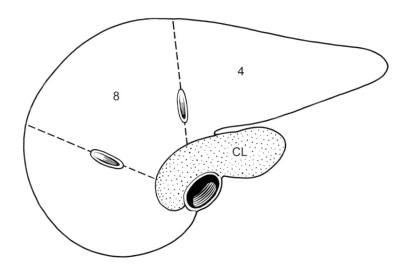

There is a proper caudate vein that drains directly from the caudate into the left side of the vena cava; it is rarely visible. On the right side a caudate process vein drains into the right IVC and is often taken when mobilizing the right liver off the inferior vena cava.

➢ **Wisdom**

You cannot classify the caudate; you have to know it.

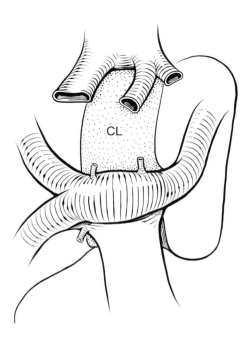

Hepatic veins and inferior vena cava

There are really only two hepatic veins outside the liver. The middle and left hepatic vein are almost always a common trunk that bifurcates within the parenchyma. There is a very useful space between the right and middle hepatic vein that can be used to dissect either way or straight down on the top of the vena cava. It is essential to remember that dissection planes around the hepatic veins always follow the surface of the vena cava. On the left, the path around the trunk ends in a space just above the tip of the caudate. On the right, the path around the vein comes up against the IVC ligament.

The hepatic veins do not have a sheath and are in direct contact with liver parenchyma. During dissection these are the structures that bleed. Unlike sheaths, there are hepatic vein collaterals between sectors and segments; dividing a major hepatic vein does not cause the liver to swell or blow up as long as the other major veins are intact. It is, however, always nice to preserve as many hepatic veins as possible.

It is an underappreciated fact that the liver encircles the upper inferior vena cava in a fashion. The posterior aspect of this encirclement is usually a ligament between segment 7 and the caudate lobe but it can occasionally be composed entirely of liver tissue. In other words, the Spiegel lobe surrounds the IVC (20% of livers). This 'IVC ligament' is important when doing right hepatectomies. It is also known as the hepatocaval ligament or the dorsal ligament.

➢ Wisdom

The upper inferior vena cava is encircled by liver/IVC ligament.

The inferior vena cava is intimate with a shallow depression in the back of the liver. A series of hepatic veins enter on the right side. The upper right hepatic vein is usually dominant. However, separate middle and lower right hepatic veins can often be found extending from the right side of the liver into the vena cava. There are few tributary veins between the centre of the

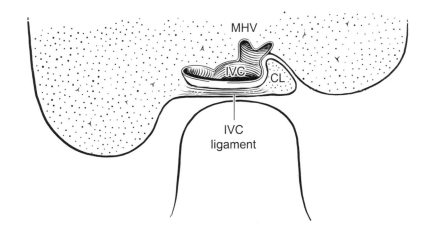

IVC and the liver; this avascular space can be readily opened. There are posterior (dorsal) venous tributaries into the vena cava, including adrenal, suprarenal and phrenic vein branches. They are important to understand in vascular exclusion techniques.

The inferior vena cava can be exposed for a short area below the liver and above the renal veins. This may require moving the porta hepatis to the left and taking the peritoneum off both left and right sides. It is a useful emergency control point for liver bleeding by clamping the IVC to reduce venous pressure within the liver.

Wisdoms

- *First get oriented and then get operating.*

- *The liver is separated by oblique irregular planes into odd-shaped segments.*

- *The hilar plate is the entry point for key moves into the liver.*

- *Glissonian 'vasculobiliary' sheaths are the end units to each liver area.*

- *The three sectors of the liver are anatomically consistent.*

- *One sheath, one segment, is a myth.*

- *The umbilical fossa is a rare anatomic gift to the centre of the left liver.*

- *You cannot classify the caudate; you have to know it.*

- *The upper inferior vena cava is encircled by liver/IVC ligament.*

Chapter 14

Liver procedures

It is a characteristic of wisdom not to do desperate things.
Henry David Thoreau

Operating on the liver should never be taken lightly. It is surprising how quickly events can spiral out of control once one enters the parenchyma. 'Chip shots' are the exception. An extensive knowledge base of internal liver anatomy and real time experience with a cadre of mentors is essential. An HPB surgeon must have internalised a quiver of techniques that can be applied strategically to forge the operative pathway with the best outcome. The landscape is variable and the path is unpredictable.

 Wisdom

Liver operations follow an unpredictable and changeable path.

Making a liver operative plan

High-quality imaging remains the foundation of all liver surgery. Tumor board meetings to review images (face-to-face conferencing) with a radiologist experienced in HPB imaging is a quality indicator for any HPB program. It is surprising how often new or insightful pearls are put on offer during these meetings. It provides you with a nuanced understanding into the sometimes uncertain nature of radiologic interpretations. Magnetic resonance (MR) studies have become the lynchpin of all liver imaging. This sophisticated technique can usually give a reasonable 'pathological' diagnosis to any liver mass. The need for biopsy is rare and even when some uncertainty exists, a little watchful waiting can document concerning growth. Liver biopsies are mostly needed to plan chemotherapy in the borderline resectable or palliative situation. While you may be an expert in the interpretation of computed tomography (CT) images, MR imaging is becoming increasingly complicated with multiple sequences and different contrast agents. Preoperative review will assure that, in the operating room, you know which sequences are important and where to look. Contrast-enhanced ultrasound and CT positron emission tomography (PET) imaging may also be useful adjuncts.

➤ Wisdom

Get to know your liver radiologists... well.

Based on clear CT or MR imaging, a preoperative plan for resection is crucial. As the years have passed, surgeons have moved to more parenchymal-sparing procedures and therefore, perform fewer extended resections where morbidity and mortality are higher. More importantly, however, the quality of liver surgery is often dependent on margin status; limited resections with positive margins represent all risk and no benefit. Central lesions and lesions near proximal hepatic veins usually require a major hepatectomy. Anything near the surface can be removed with non-anatomic segmental resections. The true removal of an anatomic segment is a good thing and should be completed when possible; however, we more often pretend that this is what we do. Unfortunately, colorectal liver metastases and hepatocellular cancers rarely confine themselves to a single segment dashing our segmental anatomy framework.

➢ Wisdom

The quality of liver surgery is defined by margins.

Strategies for liver resection for colorectal metastases have changed in recent years. Surgeons used to count metastases; 3 or 4 representing the limit for resection. Modern HPB surgeons search for a liver zone that is metastasis free and then resect around that zone until all cancer has been removed. In many cases, that zone ends up being the caudate and segment 4. This can involve downstaging with chemotherapy, growing future liver remnants with portal vein embolization (PVE) and/or staged resections. A laparoscopic resection to clear a 'lobe', PVE and then major hepatectomy is often a good plan. The creativity of the team can be challenged by a myriad of differing metastatic patterns. The liver surgeon plays a central role in solving these complicated challenges; coordination and teamwork are essential to make the pieces of the puzzle come together.

The final decision regarding the feasibility of liver surgery often revolves around the size of the future liver remnant (FLR). A rule of thumb is 20% in normal liver, 30% post-chemotherapy and 40% for cirrhosis. As a reality check, most HPB surgeons do not like to get close to these numbers. Portal vein embolization offers an increased margin of safety by growing the FLR. It is usually well tolerated but does carry the risk of embolization material spill over into the remnant vein both prior to, and during the operation. PVE also results in hyperarterialization of the lobe. We try to avoid segmental resections in these lobes because of a perceived increased risk of bleeding.

➢ Wisdom

Be conservative with your future liver remnant plans.

ALPPS procedures (associated liver partition and portal vein ligation for staged hepatectomy; whew!) produce a more rapid growth of the FLR. This technique is utilized in an undersized FLR. The surgeon does the parenchymal dissection and ties off the portal vein to the lobe to be resected leaving it only on arterial inflow. A reoperation is then performed to complete the resection in 1-2 weeks after the remnant has grown. From an anatomic standpoint, it makes little sense that the parenchymal division enhances FLR growth greater than just PVE. Glissonian sheath collaterals between sectors do not occur so parenchymal division should not change anything of relevance after the portal vein is ligated. Compromising some arterial inflow or perhaps the hormonal stress response to surgery may be the true underlying reason for the more rapid FLR growth observed. To date, these procedures have proven quite morbid so careful consideration is mandatory. The true need for ALPPS is hotly debated. In the context of a mature liver interventional group, which can embolize segment 4 to ensure the best possible post-procedural parenchymal hypertrophy, it may not be necessary. Perhaps double hepatic vascular embolization of the portal and hepatic vein offers a safer alternative to get rapid FLR hypertrophy.

Cirrhotic patients with hepatocellular cancers (HCC) require special consideration. Segmental resection remains the rule for most patients with cirrhosis, however, a patient with a large dominant cancer in one lobe and good synthetic function can usually tolerate a hemihepatectomy. PVE offers some added safety in these cases. PVE can also be a test of how the liver and patient will behave after a resection (preoperative stress test). If the patient does not do well with PVE, they will do worse with resection. Do not attempt to resect cirrhotic patients with varices, ascites or severe thrombocytopenia!

Disappearing metastases further complicate our field of endeavour. As chemotherapy continues to improve and neoadjuvant regimes become more common, this will become an increasing challenge. To date, areas where the metastasis disappeared typically still possess viable cancer cells. As a result, if cure is the intent, they should still be resected. The placement of metallic markers by an interventional radiologist — fiducials (just like your financial advisor) — help mark these areas for future resection.

Increasingly, surgeons are combining liver and colon resections to reduce the global morbidity of two large operations. These decisions can be quite complicated and must include the consideration of both the comorbidity and frailty of the patient. In general, most surgeons will only combine limited hepatectomies (segmental or left) with large colon surgeries and large hepatectomies (right liver) with smaller colon operations on the right. The reason for the increased morbidity is not clear but may involve the elevation in portal pressure following a major hepatectomy affecting blood flow and healing in a colon anastomosis. Edema of bowel may predispose to leakage at any connection. Although Pringle maneuvers are being utilized less frequently, any necessary application before, during or after a colon anastomosis may affect the safety of bowel healing. A planned colostomy rather than an anastomosis allows for more aggressive liver surgery. Developing a preoperative plan with your colorectal colleague is useful. Of course, the liver surgeon should always go first! Liver inflow (portal vein) occlusion above a fresh colon anastomosis makes me shiver.

 Wisdom

Have a surgery plan even if you know you are going to be punched.

Incision

Choosing an appropriate incision for the planned operation can make a big difference in the conduct of the procedure. As the incision is a major source of postoperative morbidity, size does matter. Left liver resections can often be done through an upper midline incision (if not laparoscopically). This can also include low BMI patients having right liver resections. Most right liver resections require something more substantial. A simple right subcostal incision will often suffice for right segmental resections.

Anytime an incision crosses or uses the midline we have a tendency to remove the fatty falciform ligament. This can be extended up and over the liver and permanently improves access and exposure.

Larger resections require some type of flap incision, from a midline superior extension of a right subcostal incision or a Mercedes incision to an upper quadrant L incision. All flap incisions take tissue from the abdominal wall and rotate it up above the costal margin. This improves the operative space necessary for surgery under the diaphragm. Patient size and body habitus play a role in this decision with large deep cavity men often requiring the most 'flap'. A large reversed L incision provides the most exposure for a right hepatectomy. For patients having a combined colon/liver resection, an extended midline incision can provide very adequate exposure for any type of liver surgery. For truly massive and complicated resections, with caval involvement, a median sternotomy offers remarkable exposure and blood vessel control.

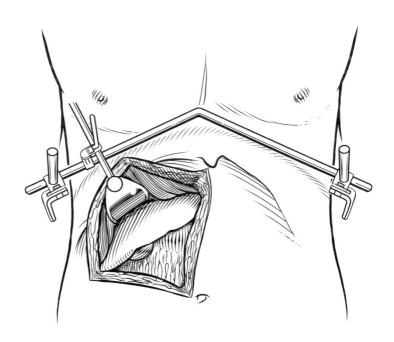

Avoiding some of these larger incisions is perhaps the biggest reason to pursue a laparoscopic approach. The thoracoabdominal incision is now mostly a historical anomaly from an older era where good abdominal wall retractors were absent.

 Wisdom

The bigger the patient, the bigger the flap incision.

Retractors

It can be argued that the two-posted (or more) retractor fixed to the operating room table has been the biggest recent advance in HPB surgery. The body and mind of a *Homo sapiens* assistant, holding a retractor, is incapable of providing the needed exposure over many operating hours. Despite some of our fondest stories, the use of students as prolonged retractor holders should be considered 'abuse' and is no longer tolerated by medical school deans. The fixed metal retractor does not complain, does not require a break and tends towards silent obedience. The first job of a trainee is to know proper retractor set-up and blade placement. Until this is mastered, little other teaching/learning can occur. For liver surgery to be successful the costal margins must be pulled up and out. Only a retractor fixed to the table can serve this purpose. The continuous readjustment of the fixed retractor blades, moving the wound opening to various points of exposure, is an art. Applying the appropriate quiver of retractor blades in strategic locations is not intuitive and must be learned from an experienced mentor.

Wisdom

Your retractor system is your loyal non-complaining partner.

Liver quality and resection

Modern life, vices and non-operative treatments all seem to be assaulting the integrity of our patients' livers. Metabolic syndrome causes liver fat, inflammation and scarring; each can affect postoperative liver function. Every patient has their own idiosyncratic response to our new chemotherapy regimens. Steatohepatitis and sinusoidal obstruction syndrome, or a combination thereof, can reduce the functional reserve of the liver. Even after waiting 4-6 weeks there is always some degree of uncertainty in regards to how the liver will function after a significant resection. A blue and mottled liver that appears friable on dissection does not enhance a surgeon's confidence. A conservative approach is always best. The procedure can be staged or the portal vein embolized to allow a margin of safety. Postoperative liver failure can torture the patient and the surgeon for months; and then end poorly.

Intraoperative ultrasound

The plan made preoperatively must be superimposed on the reality of what is found at surgery. It is surprising how often discordant findings occur. The tumors may have grown. Their location may not be as perceived on preoperative imaging. Remember that mobilization changes liver orientation. There may be new lesions and the future liver remnant may not be as large as anticipated. Real time ultrasound of the liver clarifies many of these issues. An HPB surgeon must develop the ultrasound skill to navigate the inside of the liver and understand the appearance of the different lesions and their relationship to the hilum and surrounding sheaths and veins. This allows real-time placement of the target within the liver space. This process may consume precious operating room time and mandate the assistance of colleagues including radiologists on occasion. Having a predetermined protocol for completing ultrasound assessments that survey all areas of the liver is critical and requires significant patience.

 Wisdom

Intraoperative ultrasound updates all past imaging.

Exposure, inflow control, outflow control (EIO)

You cannot cut something until you can see it. The whole process of exposure during an operation often goes by silently. A trainee not paying attention will miss these critical moves and only find this out when they are operating on their own. Pay attention and try to make yourself an operating field and not an operating pit.

➤ Wisdom

Operating in a deep hole is full of horrors.

When operating on the liver, the EIO principle is central. It stands for Exposure, Inflow control and Outflow control. No matter what you are doing, being able to easily see the structures you are operating upon is essential. Exposure starts with positioning the patient on the table. This could be as simple as moving the patient into a reverse Trendelenburg position, or as extreme as a flank approach. Let gravity help you with the operation.

➤ Wisdom

Make gravity work for you — position your patient.

The incision must be large enough and the retractors placed strategically enough to allow you to visualize all you need to. Exposure is something a surgeon is always working at, even in the late stages of an operation. The retractor system needs to be intermittently worked and then reworked as the operation moves from one area to another. New blades, moving blades and stretching abdominal wall in different directions makes visibility in different areas possible. It does not just happen and it does not just happen once. Exposure is also an approach that stresses wide dissection. When a plane is opened the structures require assessment from end to end (or side to side). If something happens at the bottom of a deep hole, everything that is critical disappears in a cauldron of blood.

 Wisdom

Exposure is an ongoing process.

Inflow control can be easily obtained by the tightening of a Rumel tourniquet around the porta hepatis. This Pringle maneuver can be used for up to an hour continuously but is more often applied intermittently with 15 minutes of occlusion, followed by 5 minutes of reperfusion. Low CVP anesthesia has dramatically reduced the necessity of the Pringle in controlling blood loss. Ischemic damage caused by inflow occlusion in a cirrhotic or post-chemotherapy liver adds another degree of uncertainty to postoperative liver function that most surgeons would like to avoid.

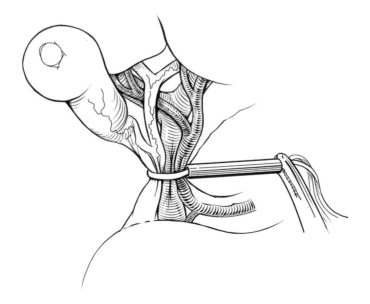

Outflow control is more challenging. During parenchymal dissection most bleeding arises from damage to hepatic vein tributaries. These veins are vulnerable as they are delicate and are not covered with a fibrous Glissonian sheath. The amount of bleeding is directly proportional to the level of the central venous pressure. A level less that 5cm H_2O is the goal.

➤ Wisdom

Bleeding comes from the pressure in the hepatic vein.

Make anesthesia your low CVP friend.

Control of hepatic veins and total vascular exclusion (TVE) techniques are now less frequently employed. They are still important for tumors at the junction of the inferior vena cava and hepatic veins. It is important to understand that despite inflow and outflow occlusion with an upper caval or hepatic vein clamp, high venous pressures in the liver may still exist. Systemic venous tributaries (adrenal and phrenic veins) are still connected and will transmit the elevated lower body venous pressures through the vena cava caudate lobe and into the liver proper. A seemingly paradoxical increase in bleeding may occur. It is important to divide all posterior venous tributaries between upper and lower vena cava clamps in TVE procedures. It is also crucial to make an early decision if TVE is going to be utilized as volume loading may be necessary to support blood pressure. TVE is not tolerated as well as a Pringle maneuver and clamp time must be kept to a minimum. Do a large part of your parenchymal dissection before clamping.

Isolated clamping of the vena cava below the liver is effective in controlling dissection plane blood loss. This maneuver immediately reduces central venous pressure and results in depressurization of the liver parenchyma. It is reasonably well tolerated (perhaps because of collaterals through the iliac-vertebral system). Systemic blood pressure support is occasionally necessary. Concurrent aortic clamping is rarely required outside the context of a hypovolemic patient suffering a significant traumatic liver smash. We routinely expose the inferior vena cava below the liver for EMERGENCY clamping if bleeding becomes problematic. Patients that have been 'overresuscitated' by an anxious anesthetic colleague can have their CVP quickly reduced with this technique. At a meeting in the early 2000s, Jacques Belghiti showed a video of a hemorrhaging middle hepatic vein during liver resection. He then clamped the IVC below the liver. It stopped bleeding — eureka!

➢ **Wisdom**

Expose the lower vena cava for clamping and quick CVP control.

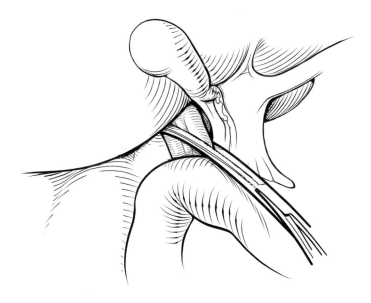

Mobilizing the right liver

Anytime we are operating on the right liver, mobilization out of the deep subdiaphragmatic cavity is necessary. Even though this is but a preliminary dissection, in a large deep person it can be quite difficult. An inexperienced assistant can easily tear the liver parenchyma, making exposure difficult as bleeding obscures the dissection plane. As more traction is applied, more tearing and bleeding may occur. Best not to get into this cycle by underestimating the importance of the mobilization process. Difficult mobilizations require an experienced assistant with a sense of just how hard to pull and direction. The liver is pulled up out of the subdiaphragmatic space. The attachment of the peritoneum on the inferior part of the liver has been called the 'rooky ligaments' as generations of students continue to pull too hard and tear the liver here. Alternating the dissection between the right lateral liver edge and the inferior edge is often an excellent strategy. When one side becomes challenging, it may be time to switch to the other; perhaps moving in a cyclical manner.

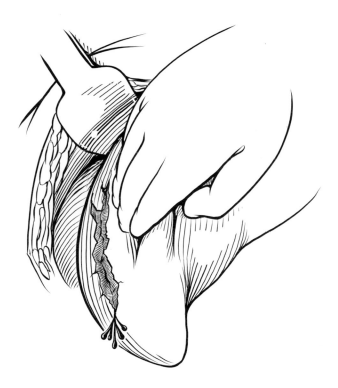

It is important to recognize that we are rotating the liver on its IVC axis; the left liver needs to go down for the right liver to come up, otherwise the liver will fold and restrict rotation. Making the dissection complete to the IVC and taking down all the attachments of the left will allow this maximum mobilisation to occur. The right adrenal gland can occasionally be fused to the posterior liver and require some careful dissection to prevent bleeding.

➤ Wisdom

Tearing the deep right liver during mobilization causes tears.

IVC and hepatic vein dissection

The inferior vena cava is your friend. It is a thick-walled vein with (hopefully) low pressure. Extending the dissection to remove the caudate from the inferior vena cava is usually straightforward. Moving up towards the right hepatic vein facilitates encircling this vein on top of the cava. The IVC ligament generally gets in the way and should be divided. We use small clips as they are less likely to rub off; this also controls the small vessel that is usually found behind the ligament itself. Also, the 'ligament' can occasionally be composed completely of liver tissue, encircling the upper IVC and connecting with the caudate on the left side. A difficult ligament can be divided with an endoscopic stapler (vascular load).

It is often not well recognized that when the right liver is completely mobilized, the IVC ligament is pulled anteriorly. This can kink the IVC, cause decreased venous return and hypotension. Tell your agitated anesthetist to have a nap and then proceed with dividing the ligament. It can be a little disorienting to think that pulling the liver up compresses the vena cava unless you know some anatomy!

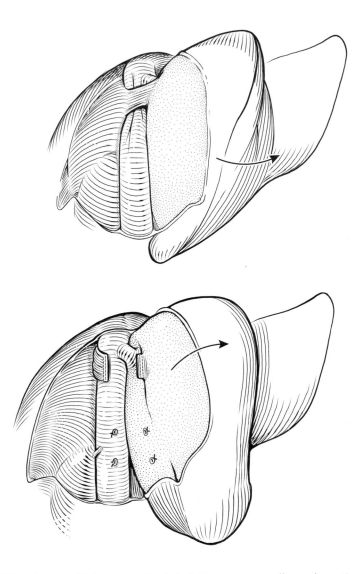

It has been widely recognized that there are usually no hepatic venous tributaries in the central space above the vena cava. Right hepatic veins, of which there can be several (superior, middle and inferior), originate from the right side of the IVC and there is a large caudate vein on the left. This leaves a central space that can be dissected by starting between the right and middle hepatic veins. Most of this dissection is done from below, proceeding superiorly parallel to the cava. This dissection is required for safe right hepatic vein encirclement. By passing a large right angle dissector down the space between right and middle hepatic veins, it is possible to connect with the inferior dissection and allow a tape to be pulled through and then around the right hepatic vein. The direction of this dissection is parallel to the vena cava.

➢ Wisdom

The centre of the retrohepatic vena cava is empty.

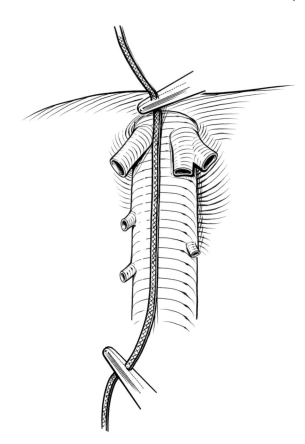

Dissection of the trunk of the middle/left hepatic vein can be useful for control of these veins when tumors are located in the superior parts of segment 4a or 2. This involves dissecting around both left and right sides of the trunk. On the left, the space above the caudate on top of the vena cava is developed. You sometimes have to divide the ligamentum venosum in this space. The area under the middle hepatic vein is opened and these two areas of dissections are connected. It is important to recognize that the direction is transverse and runs over the top of the vena cava. It cannot be forced. The middle or left hepatic veins can be isolated individually, but this requires more effort and is riskier as the dissection often descends into the liver parenchyma.

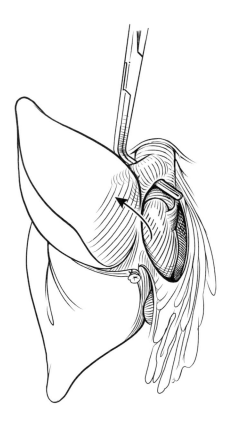

Removing liver segments

When removing parts of the liver, three-dimensional thinking is essential. There are very few reliable landmarks as parenchymal dissection extends deep into the liver. It is very easy to become spatially disoriented and end up in the wrong plane, effectively 'lost in space'. This is especially true in the right liver (right hepatectomy or extended left hepatectomy). Using the intraoperative ultrasound to mark out the margins of the tumor before starting can be useful and prevent the horrible feeling of finding oneself face to face with the tumor wall. This should be done after mobilization, however, as the orientation will change. The middle hepatic vein can be a useful landmark of the midhepatic plane (main portal fissure).

Lesions around the periphery and towards the surface can be removed by segmental resection. This is rarely a true anatomic segment. On the left side, going after proximal Glissonian sheaths is reasonable as they are accessible on either side of the umbilical fossa. However, on the right, the sheaths are deep and inaccessible unless a significant amount of parenchyma is first divided. Because they arise deep to the surface, a better strategy is to divide the branches as they are encountered. Segmental resection is, however, still an anatomic principle that guides resection and preserves vascularized parenchyma. The deeper the lesion, nearer to proximal sheaths (hilum) and hepatic veins, the less viable 'segmental' resection becomes. Eventually a lobe or sector has to come out; margins count.

Segmental resections must be planned with care; starting wide and coming around the deep margin, well away from tumor. Starting too close to the tumor compromises margins and creates a vertical hole which always bleeds at the bottom. Use your ultrasound to know where the tumor, sheaths and veins reside. Use cautery to mark out your resection on the surface of the liver, but only after you have completed your ultrasound survey. The cautery marks will obscure the ultrasound image. There is no point in leaving a large area of devascularized liver so if you need to take a larger sheath be sure to include the downstream liver in your resection. Stay sutures in the segment to be removed and even in the surrounding liver allow gentle traction to separate the resection plane and provide good visibility.

Wisdom

Go wide for segmental resections.

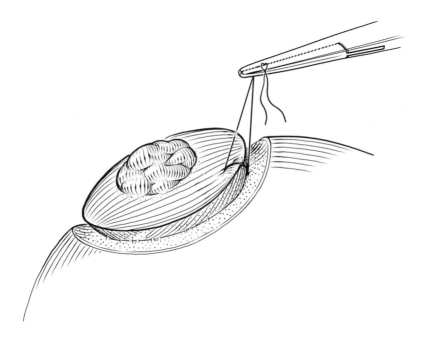

Removing liver 'lobes'

Taking out a lobe of the liver is really code for a hemihepatectomy; the term 'lobe' is a bit of a misnomer. Hemihepatectomies involve significant parenchymal dissection and central sheath division. There are three ways to divide inflow to the hemi-liver being removed: 1) subhilar with individual ligation of artery and vein; 2) primary Glissonian sheath division; or 3) sheath division during parenchymal dissection. This is largely a matter of personal choice.

It is possible to detach the hilum from the liver and bring it out into the light of day. Connecting dissections under segment 4 and around the hilar plate to a posterior dissection through the caudate process will make this happen (the posterior approach). This approach was developed by Bernard Launois in France and exposes a window to the central liver and sectoral sheaths on the right.

➤ Wisdom

The hilar plate is the window to the central liver.

It is often satisfying to divide inflow to the planned resection side and watch the liver demarcate at the start of the procedure. It can limit blood loss during parenchymal dissection. During right hepatectomy, dissecting the porta and individual ligation of the hepatic artery and portal vein is a useful exercise to familiarise surgeons to the dissection under the hilar plate (a requirement for hilar tumor resection). It may also improve safety by defining the central bile duct location. While we divide the right hepatic artery, we often only tie the right portal vein. This usually avoids the troublesome short caudate vein in this area. It can be challenging to orient a stapler in this compact area. With this technique we eventually definitively staple the right Glissonian sheath to divide the plate, bile duct and vein.

It is important to know that there may be two, or rarely more, right portal veins (separate right sectoral veins) and more than one right hepatic artery. It is crucial to clearly identify and preserve the vessels to the remaining left

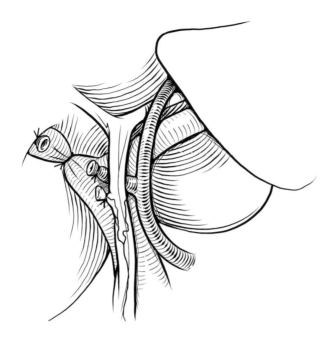

liver. Dissect the bifurcation, clamp the discovered veins and check demarcation. Check hepatic artery pulsation on the left side of the porta hepatis. There is a rare anatomic abnormality where there is a single inflow Glissonian sheath to the entire liver with no hilar bifurcation.

➤ Wisdom

Be sure of the blood flow to your remnant liver before any blood vessel division.

When removing the right liver, it is also possible to damage the central bile ducts at the hilar plate, where they bifurcate left and right. The Glissonian sheaths in the right liver arise from a short common trunk that widens out quickly to form the right anterior and posterior sheaths. This can force the surgeon's dissection centrally where a staple line may include the bile duct bifurcation. Get oriented before firing the stapler. Taking the anterior and posterior sectoral sheaths separately on the right is an option that can improve safety.

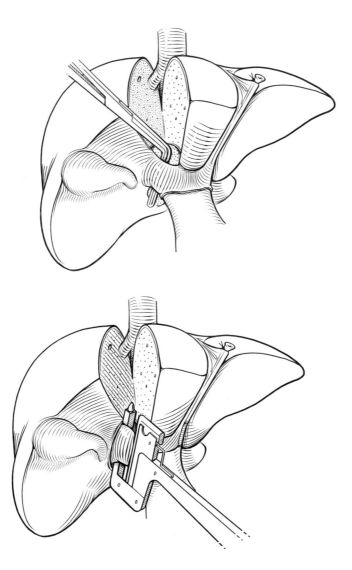

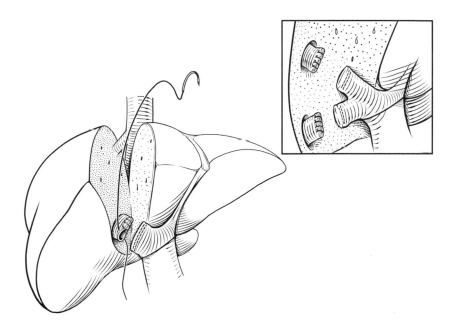

With right hepatectomies, keeping the parenchymal dissection on the correct plane can be difficult. We divide the right hepatic vein with an endostapler and completely dissect the IVC and caudate apart before the parenchymal dissection. This enhances directional control by allowing the operator to move straight down onto the vena cava. It also makes completion of the posterior part of the operation easier. With the vena cava pre-dissected, several fires of a linear stapler can quickly and safely complete the operation without any risk of damaging vena caval tributaries. The posterior part of the dissection moves through the right side of the caudate.

Dissection of the right sectoral sheaths may also cause the operative plane to wander off into the right liver rather than straight down onto the cava. To prevent this, we often place a vertical tape on top of the cava around the whole liver and use it to guide our downward dissection. The tape acts as a surrogate landmark. The major risk of getting lost in the right liver is unnecessary blood loss from too much parenchymal dissection and leaving a lot of devascularized liver post-resection.

➤ Wisdom

Use all your landmark tricks to prevent getting 'lost in space'.

When stapling hepatic veins, it is important to note the appropriate direction of the staple line. On the right hepatic vein, the direction of the staple line is vertical and on the middle left hepatic vein trunk, it is horizontal. If you mix this up you may have to watch your staple line 'unzip', an unpleasant experience.

➤ Wisdom

Know what direction to staple the hepatic veins.

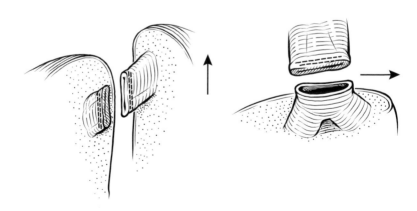

Right liver resections can be divided into three components: the upper parenchyma, the right Glissonian sheath(s) and the posterior aspects (caudate). It's nice to divide a large amount of parenchyma over the top of the liver before heading deep into the more risky central liver. Packs behind the right liver hold it horizontal. When the sheaths have been divided it may be useful to remove the packs and allow the right liver to drop posteriorly. This exposes the deep line of dissection above the vena cava. A finger or tape within the plane above the cava defines this last part of the dissection line.

Central bile ducts going into the liver first follow plates and then sheaths. You do not find a bile duct alone within the parenchyma. At the main biliary bifurcation, the bile ducts may form a trifurcation (11%) and not infrequently a right sectoral duct can cross over from the main left bile duct (9%). In a left hepatectomy it is theoretically possible, with central division of the hilar plate, to divide a sectoral duct to the right liver. To avoid this, we divide it further left under the umbilical fossa.

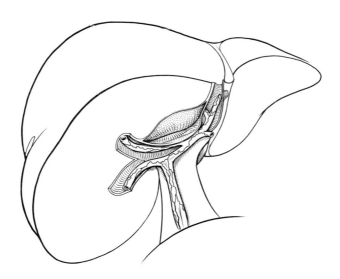

Instead of a single left hepatic duct, there may be two or more left bile ducts in the hilar plate. Central biliary abnormalities largely go unrecognized when we divide plates and sheaths. It does, however, become important in biliary reconstruction after hilar cholangiocarcinoma resections.

Left hepatectomies can start with a subhilar dissection of the left portal vein and left hepatic artery as on the right. However, it is somewhat easier on the left to divide the entire inflow by controlling the vasculobiliary structures en masse under the umbilical fossa. This maneuver is more accessible on the left side than the right. The dissection goes over the left side of the hilar plate and into the caudate lobe proper. A vessel loop is then passed to guide placement of the linear stapler.

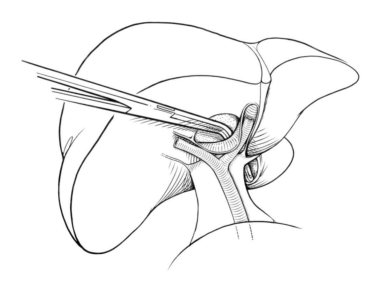

Anatomic landmarks for left-sided resections are not the same as for right-sided resections. The caudate lobe does not usually need to be removed.

This means that the vena cava cannot be used as a posterior landmark. The dissection plane goes down the main portal fissure with the middle hepatic vein employed as a good landmark. The right liver is not mobilized, as for a right hepatectomy, so the direction of this dissection, along the same mid-plane, is at a completely different angle (oblique and angled right to left). At some undefined level, the surgeon must sense where the caudate lobe is located and dissect left over the top of it. It is easy to get lost. The posterior hilar plate and path of the ligamentum venosum (LV) can help with orientation to the appropriate level. We try to leave the middle hepatic vein unless the tumor is close. We also rarely divide the middle left hepatic vein trunk prior to parenchymal dissection. The space here is small for an endoscopic stapler and the left hepatic vein can be taken nicely with a linear stapler as a last step in the operation.

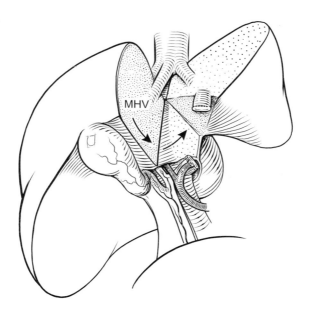

During extended left hepatectomies, surgeons are prone to spatial disorientation. The middle hepatic vein landmark is absent. The midspace in the right liver is effectively featureless. The right hepatic vein between the right anterior and posterior sectors is quite deep. Go slow and orient back to the hilar plate and extrahepatic origin of the right and middle hepatic vein. When doing any extended resections, the future liver remnant is drained by only one hepatic vein. The dissection often comes close to this vein. Extra care is needed as this structure cannot be damaged and then narrowed with sutures!

Resection of segments 2/3 (left lateral sectionectomy) is a great 'starter' hepatic resection — open or laparoscopic. The parenchyma is relatively thin and the umbilical fossa shows the way. The dissection plane should be to the left of the fossa to prevent damage to the central portal vein. There is also an 'umbilical' branch of the left hepatic vein that runs in the plane above the umbilical fossa.

➢ **Wisdom**

Segment 2/3 resection is a great starter hepatectomy.

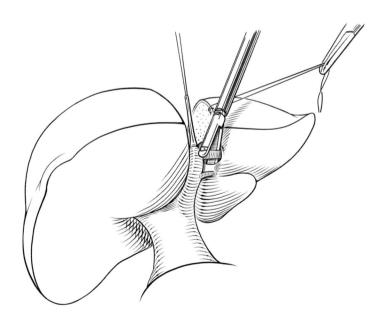

The 'hanging liver' technique is utilized for a very large right liver tumor or where diaphragm invasion makes mobilization unsafe. It is based on the anatomic absence of central venous tributaries along the retrohepatic vena cava. This space can be dissected blindly from below with a long aortic clamp and a tape can be passed through to the space between the middle and right hepatic veins. The liver is then suspended along the primary vertical partition line. The tape is a directional landmark and traction allows a modicum of bleeding control in the deep parenchyma. There is no preliminary dissection and the hepatic veins and vena cava are dissected last.

Do not think twice about resecting some of the diaphragm if the tumor is attached. Close the hole with interrupted non-absorbable sutures and suck out the air with a red rubber catheter before tying the final stitch. A positive pressure extended breath by your anesthesiology colleague will help.

Central liver issues

Central or mesohepatectomies sound more impressive than they really are. Making two major lines of parenchymal dissection adds time and risk. For more superficial central lesions, this is reasonable (segment 4b), but if the tumor is deep or near the origins of the hepatic veins it may be faster and safer to do a hemihepatectomy or extended procedure. Preoperative portal vein embolization adds safety if the future liver remnant is small.

While the hilar plate is a key anatomic structure for entry into the liver, it is also quite delicate. Using energy devices near the plate and remaining central Glissonian sheaths should be avoided. Anything that produces heat can damage vessels in the plate and central sheaths. This can include cautery, Harmonic Scalpel®, Aquamantys™, Habib®, etc. Because the bile ducts reside within these fibrous structures, they can be devascularized with any damage to the plate. This 'burn' can result in complete destruction of the central bile ducts, a devastating injury that can be impossible to repair, leaving the patient with a permanent drain and recurrent cholangitis. Switch to a blunt technique in this area, even if there is more bleeding. If you are using heated saline (Aquamantys™, TissueLink™) be sure the supraheated liquid does not pool on the hilar plate or any other structure! Your radiologic colleagues may need reminding that the use of ablation devices near the central hilar plate or proximal Glissonian sheaths is risky.

Wisdom

The central liver (hilar plate) does not like energy devices.

Caudate resection

Because of its unusual anatomy and deep location, the caudate lobe demands respect. Removal of a tumor from the left caudate (Spiegel lobe) is relatively straightforward as it hangs free on the left side of the IVC. However, a more central tumor above the vena cava is a complicated matter as this space is small and difficult to expose. The hepatic veins and the base of other segments may be involved with tumor. Resection of a cancer in this location are often combined with a hemihepatectomy. Central hilar biliary tumors often extend along caudate ducts/sheaths that exit posteriorly into the caudate proper; they require removal of some or all of the caudate to get negative margins. This scenario is ideally recognized early in preoperative imaging and planned for in advance of the operation.

Parenchymal dissection (controlling blood loss)

At the beginning everyone has a plan; bleeding is the ultimate scrambler of that plan. It destroys whatever limited anatomic clarity you may have. Liver surgery used to have such a blood-letting reputation that anesthesiologists would immediately start fluid loading the patient to anticipate massive hemorrhage. Unfortunately, this would raise the central venous pressure and guarantee massive blood loss during parenchymal dissection. Indeed, low CVP anesthesia is now universally practiced to significant effect. Blood transfusions are much less common; far less than 20% in most centers. Other strategies are also in play, including a general increased familiarity with hepatic anatomy, and better retraction.

➢ Wisdom

Bleeding is the 'Mike Tyson' of your plan.

Parenchymal dissection has also improved with newer tools. They can be divided into three groups: tools that disintegrate liver tissue to expose vessels for control (CUSA®, ERBEJET®); tools that ablate a line of liver tissue for sharp division (Habib®, Aquamantys™, TissueLink™); and tools that ablate and divide tissue (Harmonic Scalpel®, LigaSure™). It is important for trainees to become familiar with these tools and be competent with at least one. In general, they have reduced the pace of dissection with more control rather than rapid transection and packing. Whatever the technique, larger structures (hepatic veins and sheaths) must still be encircled and controlled. Cautery, clips, ties and staplers are employed for the ever-increasing size of the structure to be controlled.

Despite all these advances, the potential for massive blood loss remains. The early part of the operation, in all cases, should include wide mobilization under good exposure. A Rumel tourniquet should be placed loosely around the porta hepatis and the lower cava exposed for clamping and rapid CVP reduction, if necessary. Dissection of the hepatic veins can also allow direct outflow control. A knowledge of how to apply pressure, pack or even the use of a large liver clamp can be useful. Suture ligatures, clips, cautery and staplers need to be at the ready. Most of this has to be learned first-hand in the operating theatre as part of a mentor-driven process. It is useful to see the parenchymal division as a two-surgeon technique with one using the tool and the other using the clip applier, cautery and suction. The speed of the dissection is important. The goal is to make steady progress. Too slow and a small amount of bleeding adds up; too fast and bleeding may become excessive.

➢ Wisdom

Parenchymal division is a dance of different techniques and speed control.

You cannot say too much about cautery when it comes to controlling blood loss. The creation of an eschar plug is truly an art. Generally, the cautery must be turned up to a power level between 60 and 90 watts. Too little and the eschar does not form quickly enough and too much and all you get is sparking. Place the blade above where the torrent is arising and work your way down onto the stream. Let gravity be your friend. You must apply enough pressure for the eschar to stick to parenchyma without forcing the blade into the liver. The blade of the cautery must be clean so the eschar does not stick and pull off. A clip on the vessel may provide a very effective nidus for the eschar formation. Your mentor must show you how to do this and it must be practiced. It is important to develop a feel for when it will work and when it will not.

➢ Wisdom

Learn to make an eschar plug with your cautery.

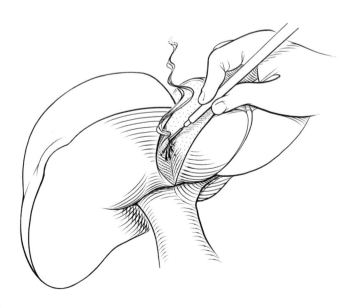

As one works their way through the parenchyma the rate of bleeding needs to be monitored and the pace of the operation adjusted accordingly. If bleeding seems to be getting out of control the first step is inflow occlusion with your Rumel tourniquet. The next step is lower caval clamping. At this point the pace of the parenchymal dissection must increase dramatically as there is a limit to the time a patient and his/her liver will tolerate this ischemia. Rarely, rapid removal with repeated staple firing and packing may be necessary to prevent a trauma type scenario. Blood loss of several liters can induce acidosis, hypothermia and coagulopathy. Knowing when to switch to damage control is a difficult skill to acquire but can certainly save a patient's life. Abandoning the procedure, packing and sending the patient to the intensive care unit is a humbling process. An early request for a colleague's help or even scheduling two surgeons for a difficult procedure is prudent and may avoid trouble. As situations deteriorate, the expertise of your assistant becomes more and more critical.

Dividing the cirrhotic liver is a different beast. Your tools will not work the same as on a normal liver. The tissues are hard and do not separate well. It is difficult to avoid making holes in the hepatic veins and they are generally more difficult to control. The fibrotic parenchyma holds these vessels open. Of course, these are just the patients who you do not wish to compromise liver with ischemia from inflow occlusion. Sometimes alternate strategies work; we often switch to a Harmonic® scalpel and suture ligatures. Prepare yourself for trouble and have a more limited set of goals.

Laparoscopic liver resection

Laparoscopic resection of part of the liver has been incorporated into the practice of most HPB surgeons. The techniques are the same as open and almost anything that can be done open can be done laparoscopically. The extent of resection that surgeons will perform is quite variable. Segmental resections along the anterior liver edge (segments 2 to 6) and segment 2/3 (left lateral sectionectomy) resections are the most common. The ambient high pressures of the pneumoperitoneum certainly does help with hepatic venous bleeding; low CVP anesthesia should still be practiced.

Proper patient position can be very helpful. Putting the patient head up gets gravity to pull the liver away from the diaphragm. Getting the ports in the right position takes some thought as being too close or too far away will hamper dissection. Transthoracic ports may be necessary for right liver resections. Large stay sutures for liver retraction can facilitate progress. For far right-sided lesions (segment 6 or 7), positioning the patient with their right side up can be very effective as gravity holds the liver away from the diaphragm for posterior exposure. Obtaining the correct angles for dissection is an ongoing process and requires practice. Once parenchyma has been thinned by using the various energy devices, endostaplers are a joy. The parenchyma is divided in layers with the energy device. Slow and deliberate work allows the device time to coagulate vessels. The tip of the device should not be forced; at any resistance it should be redirected. Intraparenchymal sheaths and veins need to be clipped or stapled.

A left lateral sectionectomy is perhaps easier laparoscopically than open. After dividing the triangular and falciform ligament a suture will provide lateral traction for segment 3. Some surgeons leave the falciform intact to maintain the liver suspended. The parenchyma to the left of the falciform is 'thinned' down to the segment 2 and 3 sheaths to the left of the umbilical plate. These can be stapled sequentially. The plate of Arantius (avascular) can be divided and the left hepatic vein can then be taken at an angle with some liver parenchyma.

Converting to an open procedure is a natural part of every laparoscopic surgeon's toolkit. Getting negative margins should not be compromised. Remember, patient first, ego second. If you start to think about conversion, communicate and move the open instruments into the room (at the very least a knife to open) while you work on control. Conversion for massive bleeding is a risky option as dropping the pneumoperitoneum releases the flood gates and open exposure may not be quickly obtainable. This can become a trauma situation. Follow your laparoscopic bleeding strategy. If your laparoscopic skill is not there yet, open well before bleeding causes hemodynamic instability. A good strategy for high-ego surgeons is to label a converted procedure, 'laparoscopically-assisted'. This gets us away from the label, 'failed laparoscopic procedure'.

 ## Wisdom

Conversions should be labeled 'laparoscopically-assisted' rather than 'failed'.

Bleeding control during laparoscopic liver procedures

Real bleeding is always a challenge in laparoscopic procedures. You need a strategy that is worked out in advance. Subhilar control of inflow vessels and hepatic vein division prior to parenchymal dissection are the same as for open techniques. For moderate bleeding, clips, bipolar cautery and unipolar electrocautery 'eschar plugs' can work. With the start of any significant bleed there is often a short window where the vessel can be seen and controlled with a grasper before the field fills with blood or the camera lens is squirted.

Inflow control with a Pringle maneuver is as viable a procedure laparoscopically as open. It decreases hepatic artery/portal vein flow directly and hepatic vein bleeding indirectly by decreasing CVP. The laparoscopic approach offers new advantages over open surgery. The pneumoperitoneal pressure can be increased to effectively dampen bleeding. A carbon dioxide embolus can certainly occur and is a concern but seems to be mostly tolerated. A short discontinuation of ventilation can also reduce venous bleeding and allow the application of a practiced technique for suture control. A suture ligature using clips at either end works for those of us who are challenged at knot tying. This 'rescue ligature' and needle driver should be always on the table and ready to go in preparation for a 'bleeding event'. A hand port can also be used to apply pressure as in open surgery.

Wisdom

Practice your laparoscopic suturing no matter what your age.

Completing a liver operation

Once you have placed that piece of liver on the table, it's 'Miller time'. NOT so fast! There is another checklist to do. First make sure it is absolutely dry. Suture it, burn it, or place magical substances on it, but do not leave it bleeding. Then make sure the bile ducts are not going to leak. The staplers are not perfect and can occasionally leave an open duct or vessel in the corners. Oversew the staple lines. Examine the parenchyma for bile and repair any leaking ducts. A clean sponge will 'show you the green'. Replace the liver in its anatomic position and suspend it if necessary. We always suture the falciform ligament to the diaphragm in a right liver resection. A torqued hepatic vein will kill your patient overnight.

Be sure you and your anesthesia colleague have a plan for returning the patient to euvolemia after hours of low CVP; acute renal failure postoperatively is common after hepatectomy. Postoperative pain control should be discussed. Oh, and by the way, how is the patient you just operated on actually doing? The first 24 hours is a critical time where serious problems often become manifest. These problems always start in the operating room.

Wisdom

Work the end of a liver operation.

Wisdoms

- *Liver operations follow an unpredictable and changeable path.*

- *Get to know your liver radiologists... well.*

- *The quality of liver surgery is defined by margins.*

- *Be conservative with your future liver remnant plans.*

- *Have a surgery plan even if you know you are going to be punched.*

- *The bigger the patient, the bigger the flap incision.*

- *Your retractor system is your loyal non-complaining partner.*

- *Intraoperative ultrasound updates all past imaging.*

- *Operating in a deep hole is full of horrors.*

- *Make gravity work for you — position your patient.*

- *Exposure is an ongoing process.*

- *Bleeding comes from the pressure in the hepatic vein.*

- *Make anesthesia your low CVP friend.*

- *Expose the lower vena cava for clamping and quick CVP control.*

- *Tearing the deep right liver during mobilization causes tears.*

- *The centre of the retrohepatic vena cava is empty.*

- *Go wide for segmental resections.*

- *The hilar plate is the window to the central liver.*

- *Be sure of the blood flow to your remnant liver before any blood vessel division.*

- *Use all your landmark tricks to prevent getting 'lost in space'.*

- *Know what direction to staple the hepatic veins.*

- *Segment 2/3 resection is a great starter hepatectomy.*

- *The central liver (hilar plate) does not like energy devices.*

- *Bleeding is the 'Mike Tyson' of your plan.*

- *Parenchymal division is a dance of different techniques and speed control.*

- *Learn to make an eschar plug with your cautery.*

- *Conversions should be labeled 'laparoscopically-assisted' rather than 'failed'.*

- *Practice your laparoscopic suturing no matter what your age.*

- *Work the end of a liver operation.*

Chapter 15

Liver special circumstances

Knowing yourself is the beginning of all wisdom.
Aristotle

Post-hepatectomy liver failure

Despite careful planning sometimes we get it wrong and there is not enough liver to maintain normal liver function following resection. At postoperative day 1, an INR greater than 2.0 raises this concern. The 50/50 definition is as good as any (50% reduction in prothrombin time/INR >1.7 and bilirubin >50mmol/L, on postoperative day 5). Liver failure is a bit of a helpless situation. Optimize everything, provide the best supportive care and wait. Giving lactulose and vitamin K makes it feel like you are doing something and can be comforting despite a lack of any real effect. Any complication, recognized or not, can push these patients over the edge. Patients may bump along for months with failure to thrive and then have a sudden event such as bleeding or infection. Because of these dramatic terminal events, sometimes the underlying cause, liver failure, is not fully appreciated. Recovery will always be significantly delayed, even beyond the normalization of INR and bilirubin levels. Patients can die several months out or have prolonged difficulty with ascites. Liver transplantation for a completely resected hepatocellular cancer (HCC) is a consideration for a patient in extremis. Some patients should have preoperative liver transplant assessment as a 'just in case' move. Transplant remains the best treatment for a patient with HCC with poor liver function.

➤ Wisdom

There is no good medical treatment for post-hepatectomy liver failure.

Ablation (radiofrequency ablation, microwave ablation) and steriotactic radiation

Whether surgeons like it or not, other modalities for treatment of solid liver tumors are here to stay. For hepatocellular cancers less than 2cm, evidence clearly supports radiofrequency ablation as a great option with significantly less morbidity. Salvage hepatectomy for recurrence of ablation-treated tumors always remains an option for well patients with reasonable liver function. For patients with more advanced cirrhosis or varices, ablation may be the only option. The results of stereotactic body radiotherapy (SBRT) are also quite promising (as shown by the results of treatment of patients who are not operative candidates). In a patient-centred universe, these new modalities should be welcomed rather than viewed as a threat. How they are incorporated into the patient care algorithm should be the subject of ongoing clinical investigation. Indeed, the method with which we utilize intraoperative ablation technology also requires careful scrutiny.

The use of radiofrequency or microwave ablation devices within the operating room is an evolving art. At this point, resection with adequate margins still offers the best opportunity for complete tumor removal and cure. Switching to an ablation device adds some uncertainty to the margins and requires three-dimensional ultrasound orientation. If you don't have that expertise, ask your radiological colleagues to come into the OR and help you out. There are certainly circumstances where resection combined with ablation are appropriate. You are still striving for clear margins.

Laparoscopic ultrasound-directed ablation offers comorbid patients a minimally invasive approach where open surgery is too risky. It may also allow safe ablation of tumors on the liver margin where hollow organs (diaphragm, heart, stomach) could be damaged by a percutaneous approach. It causes few adhesions so has the advantage of being readily repeatable. An awkwardly placed small hepatocellular cancer in a cirrhotic liver is a good indication for laparoscopic ablation. It should be noted that ablation of lesions on the surface of the liver can result in rupture and tumor seeding. Observing this with the laparoscope is an alarming event that is not often appreciated by our radiological colleagues.

Liver abscess

Surgeons used to be responsible for treating all liver abscesses. Old surgery textbooks are full of the descriptions of local approaches. This has certainly changed with the establishment of an interventional radiologist that can very effectively place a drain in almost any abscess. While in the past, biliary tract disease, appendicitis and diverticulitis were responsible for these abscesses, this is no longer the case. A whole series of unusual bugs with no specific source are now the most common cause of these liver infections. Treatment remains antibiotics for an extended period. Many of these abscesses have multiple small loculations and are impossible to completely drain. They will almost always get better without surgical debridement. Do not get sucked into premature exploration to gain 'source control'. Set the patient's and your internal medicine colleagues' expectations for a long treatment period.

Hemangiomas

Hemangiomas are the most common liver 'tumor' found on screening for abdominal pain. Many patients have upper abdominal pain from undetermined causes. Somatization is a syndrome where we feel pain in an organ or area without an organic cause. It is real pain but it is important to remember that it is a type of pain that surgery cannot cure. Because most patients with abdominal pain are likely to have torso/body imaging, any lesion in their liver can be labeled the cause. Hemangiomas are commonly present and very rarely the pain culprit. Removing them, including ones of large size, should be avoided. Rarely, a giant hemangioma may cause pain from liver capsule stretch and warrant an operation. Other benign liver tumors including focal nodular hyperplasia and large cysts may also be implicated as a source of pain.

Having lectured this point, hypocrisy reveals that we have all removed these lesions and had patients report improvements in pain. It is, perhaps, understandably hard for patients who have invested in a significant operation not to report a positive outcome, especially when they are being prodded to do so by an enthusiastic surgeon. The placebo effect is strong, but it really does not justify the risk of a major liver resection. Enucleation is performed in some centres.

 ## Wisdom

Liver hemangiomas rarely cause pain.

Benign liver tumors

Our society has now embraced routine abdominal imaging. An abdominal ultrasound for any number of unspecified reasons can identify a liver 'mass' and this always creates patient anxiety and requires an explanation. The follow along CT and MR images often show a hypervascular mass. Statistically, these are most often focal nodular hyperplasia (FNH). These are not really a tumor but an abnormal growth of liver tissue with normal parenchymal structures (bile ducts) and an enhanced arterial blood supply, etiology unknown. A central stellate scar and absence of a capsule are common. The only reason they are important is to distinguish them from hepatic adenoma and, rarely, fibrolamellar HCC. Historically, we used liver sulphur colloid (Kupffer cells uptake) or hepatobiliary iminodiacetic acid (HIDA [bile duct uptake]) scans to distinguish these lesions. MR imaging now seems capable of making a reliable diagnosis in most cases. The use of hepatocyte-specific contrast agents (functioning hepatocyte uptake) or contrast ultrasound can usually diagnose the equivocal cases. It is unusual to need a biopsy. Hepatic adenomas are important to diagnose as they have a real but low malignant transformation rate. More important is that lesions over 5cm have a propensity to bleed and should be removed. Small lesions often involute with oral contraceptive pill discontinuation.

Simple cysts and polycysts of the liver

Explaining that a small cyst of the liver is inconsequential may be boring to you but let me assure you, it is not for the patient. These lesions can create a lot of anxiety, but only rarely symptoms. Cysts occasionally rupture, bleed internally, become infected or become large enough to distend the liver capsule and cause pain. In these cases, laparoscopic unroofing and omental transposition generally works well. A benign diagnosis can be assured on pathologic examination of the cyst wall. Simple cysts have cuboidal epithelium and cystadenomas possess columnar mucin-producing epithelium. If it is a thick-walled cyst with septations, be suspicious that it may be a cystadenoma. Be sure to speak to your pathologist if there is any ambiguity as sometimes cyst wall epithelium is discontinuous. Missing a premalignant biliary cystadenoma can be a disaster.

Polycystic liver disease should be considered a surgical disease only as a last resort. Symptomatic patients with a few isolated large cysts can be improved with unroofing. Extensive unroofing of small cysts or resection should be avoided as complication rates are high. The major problem is that the anatomy of Glissonian sheaths and hepatic veins in the cystic part of the liver is unknowable. Inevitably these structures are damaged in the dissection. The other problem is that extensive unroofing exposes significant epithelium and sets the stage for intractable ascites. End-stage patients should be considered for liver transplantation.

Hydatid cysts

In today's era of increasing immigration, patients from areas of endemic echinococcal disease may present in your office. The life cycle of

Echinococcus granulosus is a great question for junior learners and makes you look 'professorial'. Any large cyst in the liver should raise the possibility of this disease. Fortunately, their radiological appearance is fairly easy to spot, with a thick wall and daughter cysts. An elevated eosinophil count and serology can help confirm the diagnosis. Many are calcified and dead so do not require intervention. Treatment with albendazole by your friendly infectious disease specialist is the best first step. Surgical treatment is resection or enucleation of the affected liver area. If the disease is too extensive, the cysts can be sterilized with hypertonic saline injections and then the endocyst enucleated. It is critical not to spill live daughter cysts into the peritoneal cavity. Pack around the operative site with hypertonic saline-soaked sponges. Percutaneous techniques are gaining more acceptance.

Biliary cystadenoma

Biliary cystadenomas are the liver's version of the mucinous cysts that occur in the pancreas or ovary. They are most common in women where they often have a characteristic mesenchymal stroma. They are also premalignant, so removal is mandatory. A cyst with a thick wall and septations should start this thought process. At presentation, a small percentage may already have an invasive cancer component. Resection with a margin of liver is the most reasonable option for lesions in either lobe. Of course, life is never this simple; cystadenomas seem to have a predilection to grow to large sizes in the central liver. This places them on the top of the hilar plate where a real margin is not possible without liver transplantation. For cystadenomas in this location and no obvious malignancy, enucleation is reasonable. Because of the mesenchymal stroma, a plane is easy to develop and a very rewarding exploration of the central liver follows. With care the cyst can be separated from hepatic veins and Glissonian sheaths in the adjacent liver. After removal, a grand view of the vein sheath internal interplay is a real treat.

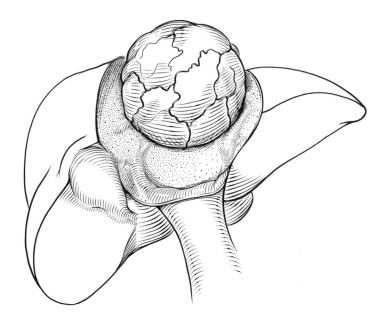

Biliary cystadenomas in men are rare, do not have mesenchymal stroma and are more likely to become malignant.

If one goes back through old surgical literature, it may be surprising to find recommendations that liver cysts be drained into a Roux-en-Y loop of small bowel. You would be wise to avoid this. Bile in the cyst fluid should not change your plans for resection. The incidence of bile leak postoperatively is increased and may require biliary decompression. Patients that have had a cyst enterostomy may present in your office. Proceed to offer them a proper operation.

➤ Wisdom

Enucleation often works for biliary cystadenomas.

Neuroendocrine liver metastases

Neuroendocrine tumors of the pancreas and carcinoid tumors of the small bowel have a propensity to spread to the liver. While surgical control of the primary lesion is a reasonable first step, the subsequent resection of liver metastases require some thought. The hormones that functioning metastases produce may cause debilitating disease. In otherwise healthy patients, removing these tumors may improve a patient's quality of life. These operations rarely cure the disease, so some moderation is reasonable. Ablations, tumor enucleation and more limited resections can be judiciously applied. Be sure to have an active octreotide infusion when you are manipulating any of these tumors.

The surgical treatment of non-functioning metastases is more controversial. These are often more aggressive tumors. Resection is reasonable with an isolated metastasis and may be useful when most of the tumor burden can be removed (>70%).

Ruptured and bleeding hepatocellular tumors

When a cirrhotic patient presents in extremis, a ruptured HCC is the diagnosis of exclusion. Unfortunately, this is how some cirrhotics present. After imaging confirms the diagnosis, be sure to send them quickly to the angiogram suite for embolization. It is amazing how effective this is! Your approach from here is less clear as rupture may have turned localized disease into disseminated peritoneal metastases. A little patient surveillance may be in order with resection or ablation down the road. Adenomas can present with bleeding in young women and when the dust settles these should be removed.

If you do end up in the operating room with a ruptured/bleeding HCC you will very quickly realize you cannot sew the ruptured bleeding porridge that you find. Better to tie off the left or right hepatic artery and call it a day. A stable patient can undergo urgent resection but then you should not be in the operating room if the patient was stable.

> ## ➢ Wisdom

The angio suite is better than the OR suite for bleeding HCCs and adenomas.

Hilar cholangiocarcinoma

A cancer could not be situated in a more difficult or hazardous location than in the hilum of the liver. In this area, snug under the hilar plate, a tumor is in contact with multiple critical structures. It is a very compact space and any real tumor extension will make resection futile or impossible. In this circumstance you will often hear the terms first-order, second-order and third-order bile ducts. First-order ducts are right and left bile ducts, second-order ducts are the two sectoral ducts on the right, and third-order ducts are segmental ducts. The implication is that tumor involvement of third-order ducts on both sides is an unresectable situation. Free first- or second-order ducts on at least one side are necessary to allow a surgical approach. Thus, in circumstances where the tumor drifts left or right, a radical surgical resection of the involved side is possible. This requires an uninvolved hepatic artery and portal vein supplying the future liver remnant. A non-regressed left or right hepatic artery that does not cross the hilum may make a radical resection possible.

MRI/MRCP seems to offer the best appreciation of the regional anatomy and should be done before any instrumentation or stenting. Cholangiocarcinomas do not show well on our present imaging modalities; delayed phase imaging may better show the extent of these tumors. Most programs prefer transhepatic stenting as it is more reliable than endoscopic stents that may be difficult to place above tumor blockage. Portal vein embolization and nutritional support are important for preparing the patient and expanding the future liver remnant for surgery. Surveillance to be sure that preoperative cholangitis is absent at the time of surgery is important. Some resectable patients never get to surgery because of recurrent obstruction and sepsis.

Liver resection often has to be extensive in these cases and include some or all of the caudate lobe as biliary tributaries/sheaths come directly off both right and left ducts. If one is taking this on, the skill to resect and reconstruct the portal vein is key. With right liver resection, the portal vein becomes redundant and will allow resection of the involved bifurcation area with an end-to-end anastomosis to the left vein. With left liver resection, reconstruction of the right portal vein is also possible with either a more limited sleeve resection or patch grafting. There is less redundancy of the right portal vein than the left in this situation. Familiarity with dissection under the hilar and umbilical plates is a critical asset. Biliary reconstruction on the right can be difficult because there are often several ducts and they may be quite deep in the liver parenchyma. Obstruction of caudate ducts may cause them to dilate significantly and necessitate their inclusion in the biliary reconstruction. In short, this is a good operation to involve two surgeons. Despite extensive surgery, obtaining a clear margin is often impossible and significant postoperative problems are frequent.

➢ Wisdom

Eat your Wheaties before attacking a hilar cholangiocarcinoma.

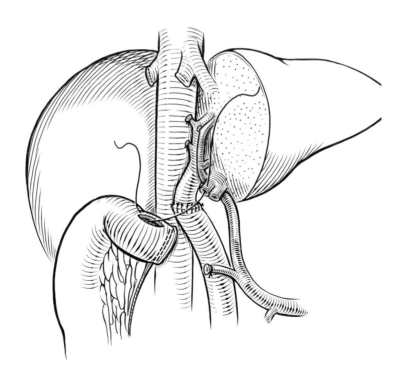

Redo hepatectomies

Staged or repeat hepatectomies for a new or residual tumor are like a bad relationship; you keep on giving and they never give back. They add a significant level of difficulty and risk. If there were any preceding postoperative leaks or infection, the level of difficulty rises dramatically. Fibrosis and scarring obscure operative planes. Count on a long pre-dissection just to get to the liver. What looks possible on CT imaging can often become a 'thrash'. After the first of a planned staged resection, wrapping the raw liver in Seprafilm® is an unproven but attractive idea to reduce difficulties in the second surgery.

Special anatomic considerations are necessary in redo hepatectomies. Compensatory growth of the remnant liver changes orientation and dissection planes. The structures of the porta hepatis can be difficult to expose under a hypertrophied remnant liver. The porta hepatis may also be rotated so that the usual three-dimensional positions of duct, artery and vein are different. In essence, our cognitive maps have to be adjusted, on the go, to accommodate these changes. Generous wide dissection with utilization of remaining landmarks, experienced assistants (second HPB surgeon) and intraoperative ultrasound will help.

Recurrent pyogenic cholangitis

There is a population of patients, mostly Asian, who have recurrent inflammation of the ducts in their liver causing fibrosis and stone formation. This disease is largely not understood and has been variably ascribed to *Clonorchis sinensis* infection. Recurrent pyogenic cholangitis (RPG) patients present with pain and recurrent bacterial cholangitis. For the most part it is not a surgical disease. However, there are a few circumstances where HPB surgeons can be helpful. Creation of a Roux-en-Y hepaticojejunostomy with an access limb allows an interventional radiologist to access ducts for stone removal and dilatation of strictures. This avoids a percutaneous approach through the liver with its attendant risks and discomfort. Some patients have disease confined to a lobe or sector. In this situation, resection of the affected area can offer real relief of symptoms. However, postoperative infection in the perihepatic space is to be expected. Chronic inflammation predisposes to cancer so all RPG patients should undergo surveillance.

Right heart failure

When the right heart does not pump adequately, the rise in systemic venous pressure immediately turns the liver into one big hemangioma. You can tell this by squeezing it and watching it compress and rebound like a sponge (just like a real hemangioma). This is a good indication to stop. Entering into a liver like this inevitably leads to a bleeding nightmare. Recognizing and medically treating heart failure may allow surgery to proceed. Repairing significant tricuspid regurgitation with valve replacement can also be an avenue to pursuing liver surgery.

 Wisdom

If the liver feels like a sponge — BEWARE.

Portosystemic shunt surgery

The creation of portosystemic surgical shunts are now largely unmentioned. It has, thankfully, completely moved into the realm of the interventional radiologist (transjugular intravascular intrahepatic shunt) and gastroenterologist (banding). Some first-generation HPB surgeons made their career on these procedures. Portocaval, mesocaval and splenorenal are all terms most young surgeons have not heard. The rare failure of non-surgical control of bleeding esophageal varices may bring this 'back to the future'. A mesocaval H graft or distal splenorenal shunt are perhaps the easiest shunt to perform and can be considered in unusual situations, but this should not be in the middle of the night. Non-shunt stomach devascularization (Sugiura procedure) and esophageal transection procedures are still options that will limit postoperative encephalopathy. An old surgical atlas may help as there are not likely to be many practitioners of these procedures left working.

Portosystemic shunts are largely historical.

Liver transplantation

Replacing a diseased liver with new has to be one of the most successful operations in history. These patients usually resume a normal life and have a near normal life expectancy. Liver transplant training is a wonderful experience for any aspiring HPB surgeon. It is an unequaled experience for learning anatomy and sewing vessels and ducts. The skill and confidence of a liver transplant surgeon translates well into routine HPB operations. Barring that, it is still important for all non-transplant HPB surgeons to understand regional and national criteria for transplant listing of HCC patients. Perhaps future options for transplantation in patients with liver only non-resectable colorectal metastases will become a realistic option in select patients. A cadre of post-liver transplantation problems may also end up in your inbox, including biliary strictures and the ubiquitous incisional hernia.

A liver transplant is the best operation.

Wisdoms

- *There is no good medical treatment for post-hepatectomy liver failure.*

- *Liver hemangiomas rarely cause pain.*

- *Enucleation often works for biliary cystadenomas.*

- *The angio suite is better than the OR suite for bleeding HCCs and adenomas.*

- *Eat your Wheaties before attacking a hilar cholangiocarcinoma.*

- *If the liver feels like a sponge — BEWARE.*

- *Portosystemic shunts are largely historical.*

- *A liver transplant is the best operation.*

Section III

Porta hepatis

The porta hepatis (hepatoduodenal ligament) deserves separate mention. It is a central part of HPB surgery and is included in almost all operations to some extent. It can also be the primary site. This small area between the liver and duodenum is packed with critical structures. While exposure is usually not a problem, biliary tumors in this area can be difficult to remove because of local vascular involvement. The interplay of the bile ducts, portal veins and hepatic arteries is complex and variable.

Chapter 16

Porta hepatis anatomy, procedures and special circumstances

Wisdom consists of the anticipation of consequences.
Norman Cousins

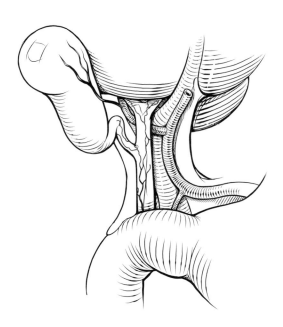

Porta hepatis anatomy

Anatomy and bile duct blood supply

The bile duct generally occupies the right side of the porta but prolonged obstruction may cause dilation that can expand it to overlay all structures. Most often the common/hepatic bile duct is straight and connects with the hilar plate before breaking into left and right branches. The right and left ducts become part of the plate and cannot be separated surgically. Duct blood supply within the plate is excellent with a fine arterial network of small vessels supplied by both right and left hepatic arteries. It is an important collateralization area for either side of the liver that loses its arterial input. Division or damage to the hilar plate will prevent collateralization from happening. The bile duct proper below the plate is not so fortunate, with a less robust axial blood supply from 3 and 9 o'clock vessels. Further, an intact duct has more of its blood supply coming from the inferior direction (60%).

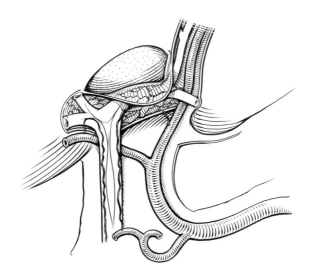

Better blood supply is why most HPB surgeons prefer the higher common hepatic duct for biliary enteric anastomoses. Further, a distal cholangiocarcinoma can extend along the duct so a higher bile duct resection margin reduces the risk of a positive margin. The closer to the hilar plate the more robust is the duct blood flow. The lower common bile duct is rarely used. Leaving tissue around the common hepatic duct is important to prevent damaging its delicate blood supply.

➤ Wisdom

Don't skeletonize the bile duct.

The proximal left hepatic duct is accessible by lifting segment 4 off the hilar plate (an anatomic point often exploited by surgeons). Most illustrations do not convey the fact that you have to get into the liver parenchyma to do this properly. This does not occur on the right side where the ducts quickly extend posteriorly into the liver as part of a Glissonian sheath. Ducts on the right are usually not accessible unless some liver tissue is removed.

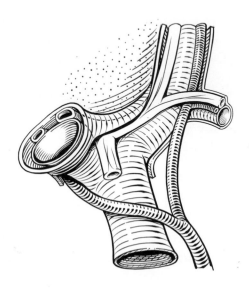

➤ Wisdom

The hilar plate and left hepatic duct are one.

The common hepatic artery is on the opposite left side of the porta and extends straight up into the umbilical fossa as it transitions into the left hepatic artery. Even if the left hepatic artery is an 'accessory' off the right gastric or coeliac axis, it still ends up in the umbilical fossa. The right hepatic artery crosses the mid-porta and usually (but not always) transits behind the bile duct. An anterior right hepatic artery (20%) may make a biliary enteric anastomosis to the common hepatic duct awkward.

During in utero embryologic development there are three hepatic arteries (right, middle and left). The embryologic right hepatic artery originates from the superior mesenteric artery, the middle from the coeliac axis and the left from the left gastric artery. In most cases, the right and left hepatic arteries regress in the porta hepatis (there is always a fibrous cord left over) leaving only the middle to become the dominant common hepatic artery. Embryologically, these three arteries all have connections within the liver through the hilar plate that persist. Non-regression may leave some or all of these arteries patent. Calling them 'accessory' or 'replaced' is anatomically confusing. Perhaps a better nomenclature would be 'non-regressed right' and 'non-regressed left' hepatic arteries. The hepatic arteries are not intimate with the hilar plate and can be dissected. The arteries are associated with a network of nerves and lymphatics that can force the operator away from the artery wall and hinders dissection. Safety with any vessel lies on the vessel wall.

The portal vein is posterior and central. It bifurcates quite high but is also not attached to the hilar plate, so can be dissected. It is also fairly robust, separates easily from surrounding tissues and is perhaps the easiest structure in the porta to encircle. Care is necessary to avoid damaging the coronary vein on the left and a superior pancreatic branch on the right.

There is also a 'parabiliary venous system' within the porta. This fine supply of venous vessels go unnoticed by most surgeons. They become important in the presence of portal vein obstruction and portal hypertension with the formation of impressive collaterals.

Porta hepatis procedures

Operating in the porta hepatis

A little time carefully reviewing the preoperative CT or MR can reveal valuable anatomic information about arteries, ducts and veins. Any operation in the porta hepatis starts with removal of the gallbladder (perhaps the only present situation where a junior resident can learn the steps of an open cholecystectomy). This improves exposure and offers access to the entire right side of the porta. The cystic duct often parallels the hepatic duct so that careful dissection can expose a good length of duct. Care must be taken not to damage the side wall of the bile duct when dissecting the cystic duct. The bile duct can then be encircled. Dissecting from left to right will prevent injury to the portal vein and staying on the bile duct wall will avoid encircling and inadvertent division of a non-regressed right hepatic artery. This artery can be palpated behind the bile duct and may be the critical blood supply to your duct. Most surgeons like to dissect the common hepatic duct with its superior blood supply. When the bile duct is divided, axial blood supply comes directly off the hilar plate. A lower connection is always complicated by the variable entry point of the cystic duct. Leaving a disconnected cystic duct stump is to be avoided. Doing a double duct anastomosis to the cystic and hepatic duct is a needless waste of time.

 Wisdom

Angle around the bile duct from left to right or suffer.

Even in a fatty porta hepatis, the pulsation of the hepatic artery is typically visible. It often takes a looping course through the bottom of the porta and can be mobilized by dividing the gastroduodenal artery. This artery is always a potential postoperative source of bleeding and requires respect. We leave a long stump that is both tied and clipped (or suture ligated). The portal vein is not difficult to dissect. It is your friend until you make a hole; it then shows you it has a high venous pressure and bleeds vigorously. Care and control of bleeding early will prevent it from spiralling out of control.

➢ Wisdom

Respect the gastroduodenal artery.

As one moves higher in the porta hepatis, the anatomy tends to increase in complexity. As dissection moves into the umbilical fossa a myriad of arteries and ducts surrounding the left portal vein are encountered. Discretion here may require operating on the other side of the umbilical plate within liver parenchyma.

Removal of the lymph nodes in the porta is usually straightforward. The large node on top of the common hepatic artery (8a) is a constant and has historically been removed for frozen section and prognostication. It may also need to be removed just to expose the area above the pancreas. The other large node posterior to the common bile duct is also often removed and may allow exposure to a non-regressed right hepatic artery. This artery is best left intact unless the right liver is being removed. A good review of the preoperative imaging should alert a surgeon to its presence. If not, it can be palpated early by feeling a pulsation behind the bile duct. Dissecting it out before dividing the posterior attachments of the pancreas will prevent injury.

The bile duct connection

Performing a high-quality hepaticojejunostomy is a premier skill for HPB surgeons. It is a part of many operations and is a connection that, in good hands, should not leak. It should not require placing a drain nearby! The principles are straightforward: no tension, good blood supply, fine interrupted sutures. A well-vascularized bile duct has the tissues around it left intact, not skeletonized. The 3 and 9 o'clock arteries can be sutured and the duct cut with a knife to avoid cautery injury, especially in a small duct. Surgeons have a habit of saying "duct to mucosa", but in reality, it is duct to everything but mucosa for most surgeons. This may be related to the original Rodney Smith jejunal mucosal graft technique of bile duct reconstruction which is only of historical interest. The opposite is now practiced; moving the mucosa out of the way is the issue. Some suture it out of the way or open the mucosa only after the back wall is completed (extramucosal hepaticojejunostomy). The anastomotic area will reendothelialize within 48 hours. If Halsted is to be believed, the submucosa is the strength layer. When making the opening in the jejunum, keep in mind that it stretches; make it just less than the inside diameter of the bile duct.

We construct our Roux limbs 50cm in length, but they probably do not have to be that long. We take extra care in dividing the jejunal mesentery. The best spot can be obtained by transilluminating the jejunal mesentery to visualize an appropriate arcade of vessels for division. The simplest and farthest apart are best. When dividing the mesentery, we can then control the crossing vessels with fine ligatures and preserve the blood supply to our bowel ends.

➢ Wisdom

*Make your bile duct anastomosis — duct to **everything but** mucosa.*

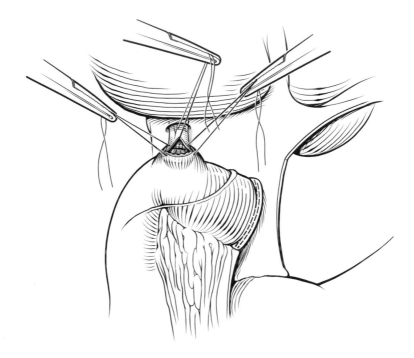

A short mesentery and/or pancreatic inflammation may make it difficult to mobilize and position the Roux-en-Y limb of jejunum next to the bile duct without tension. The most direct path is often retrocolic, through the right transverse colon mesentery just above the duodenum. Moving the Roux limb creation distally, down the small bowel mesentery, allows the limb to move more directly through this space. One should not forget that the duodenum is also there for a possible connection, in a difficult situation. The duodenum can easily be mobilized and an end-to-side anastomosis done. In a severely inflamed porta, with or without varices, a side-to-side biliary enteric connection is also a viable bail-out procedure.

Stenting of bile duct connections are not necessary in the modern era. However, if there is already a previously placed transhepatic drain we often drop it through the anastomosis. The drain can obscure visibility of the bile duct during the creation of the hepaticojejunostomy, so once we have divided the duct the 'pig tail' distal end is cut off, a silk placed through the new tip and it is pulled back into the duct. This allows the posterior wall connection to be done. It can then be easily pulled through and slid into the bowel before the anterior wall is closed. The drain skin site must be prepped and the drain resecured with a suture after the anastomosis.

As with most things, concentrating on the placement of each stitch with fine sutures (5.0 or 6.0 PDS®) and meticulous technique will produce the best results. The lumen does not have to be large for it to be functional. Significant postoperative stenosis is rare in a well-vascularized duct and only occurs after the anastomosis shrinks to a pinhole. These patients present with recurrent cholangitis and may never actually become jaundiced.

➢ Wisdom

Stents are for cardiologists, not HPB surgeons.

It may come as a surprise that the right liver may have separate extrahepatic ducts to the anterior and posterior sector (24% of patients). A low lying anterior sectoral duct is the most common (18%), followed by posterior sectoral ducts (6%). The need to reconstruct two ducts is not a rare event. If close, their medial walls can be connected before doing a single anastomosis.

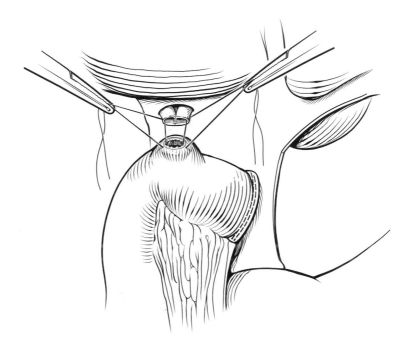

To be sure a second duct is a sectoral duct and not the cystic duct may require some probing. Separate sectoral ducts to the left liver can occur but are high at the bifurcation and not visible in the porta as they are within the hilar plate.

One of the most difficult connections occurs after left hepatectomy and hilar resection for cholangiocarcinoma. Multiple ducts deep in the right liver must be anastomosed. These ducts are often quite friable and leakage is common; it's reasonable to place an external suction drain in this situation.

➤ Wisdom

Extrahepatic sectoral ducts on the right are common. Look for them.

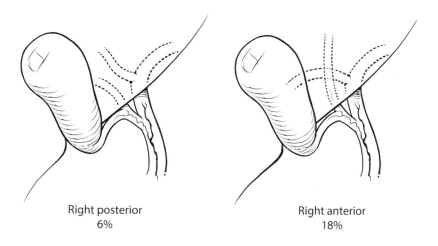

Right posterior	Right anterior
6%	18%

When doing a primary hepaticojejunostomy, forgetting to close the distal pancreatic end of the bile duct is a hazard (pancreatic head resection does not require closure as the duct is part of the resection). After you divide the duct, close the distal stump right away and you will not wake up that night in a cold sweat with a DMR — delayed mistake realization.

Porta hepatis special circumstances

Choledochal cysts (malformations)

A choledochal cyst is perhaps the biggest misnomer in all of HPB surgery. They are not cysts at all as they are not 'closed' epithelial lined cavities. Bile duct dilatations and diverticulum are perhaps more precise descriptors. Better, we should all switch to simply calling these choledochal malformations. The cyst wall is essentially the same biliary epithelium that is continuous with the rest of the biliary tree. The hallmark of these malformations is the pancreaticobiliary maljunction (PBM), present in over 90% of cases. The pancreatic duct connects with the bile duct above the ampulla creating a common channel. This may cause reflux of pancreatic fluid and predispose to malignant degeneration. These malformations can extend superiorly into the liver and inferiorly into the pancreas.

The risk of cancer and inflammation/pancreatitis are the rationale for resection. The gallbladder is also at risk and removal should be part of these operations. Resection of a choledochal malformation is the prototypical porta hepatis surgery and requires good three-dimensional understanding of the anatomy. Most of these malformations are a variation on the type I 'cyst' or fusiform dilatation. While it is often possible to remove the entire malformation, discretion can require leaving remnants of the wall behind. It is important to survey the inside of the malformation for cancer. If frozen section bears this out, a more radical cancer operation, including liver or pancreas, will be necessary to obtain negative margins. Preoperative surveillance with 'spy glass' endoscopy and biopsy may supply useful information in offering operations to elderly or comorbid patients. Indeed, a large operation in a fragile elderly patient who has had an asymptomatic choledochal malformation their whole life may not be wise. Asymptomatic 'diverticulum'-type cysts rarely become malignant and can be surveyed.

Inflammation in the cyst may result in fusion of its posterior wall to the portal vein. Leaving a layer of serosa and muscularis here will prevent injury. The inferior cuff of cyst may dive deep into the pancreatic head. It is important to avoid damage to the pancreatic duct from the PBM. While it is possible to remove much of the intrapancreatic cyst, oversewing a distal cuff may be prudent rather than a misadventure deep in the pancreas. Type 1 cysts often have separate right and left hepatic ducts entering the top of the cyst through a distorted hilar plate. Doing a complete superior cyst excision, including the hilar plate, high up in the liver, may damage the blood supply to the ducts being anastomosed. It may be safer to leave a cuff with the hilar plate intact and anastomose to this. Cancer in the proximal or distal remnants is rare (2%); the prevention of cancer is probably more related to the prevention of inflammation from pancreatic fluid reflux rather than the actual choledochal malformation resection. Lifelong follow-up is reasonable as other biliary problems such as stenosis and cholestasis may occur. Some patients may develop dilated ducts in their liver with recurrent stenosis and cholangitis that is indistinguishable from recurrent pyogenic cholangitis.

➤ Wisdom

Don't be too aggressive with either end of a choledochal cyst.

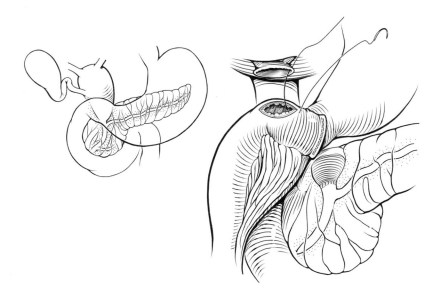

Cavernous malformation

The portal vein may clot for any number of reasons, including hereditary coagulopathies and cirrhosis. This by itself does not usually cause significant problems. Despite the name, significant portal revascularization usually occurs through the parabiliary venous plexus rather than within the vein. This results in an impressive and scary network of varices that extend around the porta and up onto the lower part of the gallbladder wall. Best to stay away. Portal biliopathy may occasionally result in biliary obstruction.

➤ Wisdom

Best to stay away from a cavernous malformation.

Wisdoms

- *Don't skeletonize the bile duct.*

- *The hilar plate and left hepatic duct are one.*

- *Angle around the bile duct from left to right or suffer.*

- *Respect the gastroduodenal artery.*

- *Make your bile duct anastomosis — duct to **everything but** mucosa.*

- *Stents are for cardiologists, not HPB surgeons.*

- *Extrahepatic sectoral ducts on the right are common. Look for them.*

- *Don't be too aggressive with either end of a choledochal cyst.*

- *Best to stay away from a cavernous malformation.*

Section IV

Gallbladder

Believe it or not, when a HPB surgery fellow graduates from HPB school they are now the gallbladder expert at their institution. Senior colleagues who have done thousands of cholecystectomies are calling for advice. The junior HPB surgeon is expected to give rounds on this subject, even though almost no extra training in cholecystectomy was done (they don't care to hear another liver talk). This demonstrates an important point: the local HPB surgeon is the community resource for gallbladder surgery and can have a great impact on patient safety.

Chapter 17

Gallbladder anatomy

Make three correct guesses consecutively and you will establish a reputation as an expert.
Laurence J. Peter

The gallbladder is a simple outpouch/diverticulum off the bile duct, so why all the fuss? Indeed, if cholesterol in concentrated bile did not have the propensity to precipitate out and form stones this section would be unnecessary. Anatomically, this sac extends under the liver; it can hang off the liver on a mesentery or be encased by liver entirely. The gallbladder location is usually under the mid-plane (main portal fissure) of the liver but it can also be found on the left or even in the umbilical fossa. It always sits on the gallbladder plate which is an extension of the hilar plate. This plate can contain small bile ducts, arteries and occasionally comes in close proximity to a large branch of the middle hepatic vein. The gallbladder plate is more attached to the gallbladder than the liver. Traction on the gallbladder will inevitably pull the plate off the liver. It leaves raw liver on the other side of the plate and it bleeds!

 Wisdom

The gallbladder plate belongs with the liver.

So how big is the gallbladder? It may seem like a silly question until one's surgical experience reveals that it can vary from filling the right upper quadrant to being the size of your thumb. Size depends on the pathologic process; this can be extremely disorienting for the surgeon who is mentally locked into a preconceived notion of size.

The hepatobiliary triangle is the critical surgical area on the right side of the porta hepatis between the common hepatic duct and the gallbladder wall. It is largely a potential space *in situ* and contains a folded cystic duct, and one or several cystic arteries. In reality it rarely forms much of a triangle. It may also contain a sectoral duct (see porta hepatis) and the right hepatic artery. The cystic artery usually runs through this area and onto the front wall of the gallbladder. It often bifurcates just before it reaches the gallbladder wall. Occasionally, the artery may be present lateral or even behind the cystic duct. The cystic duct lymph node reliably sits on the cystic artery; if it is pathologically enlarged from inflammation, it may obscure the entire triangle and even overlay the bile duct.

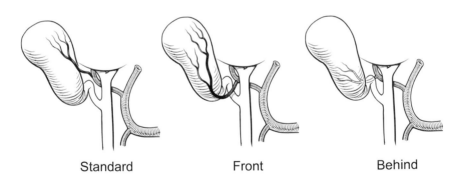

| Standard | Front | Behind |

The cystic duct is an extremely variable structure and can be long, short or non-existent (Mirizzi syndrome). It can enter the common hepatic duct high just under the bifurcation or, more often, it can parallel the common hepatic duct into the head of the pancreas. When an extra duct is encountered in the low porta hepatis it is usually this cystic duct but it is important to recognize that a right sectoral duct can look exactly the same.

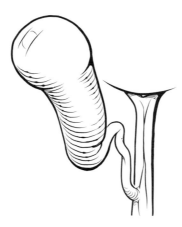

The cystic duct usually connects on the right side of the bile duct, but it may actually connect on the front, back or even cross over to the left side.

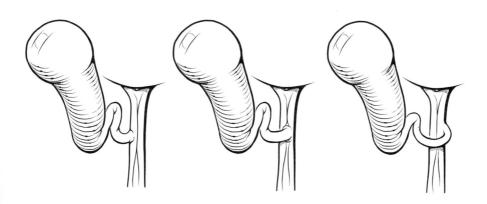

The valves of Heister can give a spiral appearance to the cystic duct but this cannot reliably distinguish it from the bile duct.

The bottom of the gallbladder is usually redundant and forms a pouch (Hartmann's pouch). This pouch often folds down below the porta hepatis but can occasionally override the entire porta hepatis. It can be found anywhere within 360° of the infundibulum (upper cystic duct).

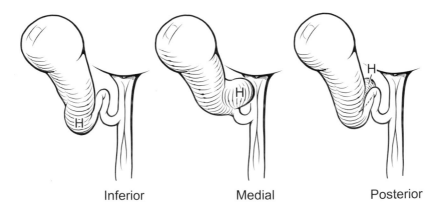

| Inferior | Medial | Posterior |

In situ, the gallbladder lays on top of the duodenum, stomach, pancreas, colon and omentum. Gallbladder inflammation can impact any of these structures. Cholecystitis can cause moderate gastric outlet obstruction! Similarly, a pathologic process in any of these surrounding organs can affect the gallbladder. Cholecystectomy may be risky in a patient with severe acute pancreatitis as the inflammatory reaction can extend around the base of the gallbladder. Varices from cirrhosis, an obstructed portal or splenic vein can course through the bottom of the gallbladder. Cancers of the colon and duodenum can invade the gallbladder and vice versa.

Everything about the gallbladder anatomy is variable. You can basically take any structure and spin it 360° around the cystic duct to determine a possible location. It is a festival of anatomic traps that lay in wait for the inexperienced or overconfident surgeon.

 Wisdom

The gallbladder is a festival of anatomic traps.

Wisdoms

- *The gallbladder plate belongs with the liver.*

- *The gallbladder is a festival of anatomic traps.*

Chapter 18

The safe cholecystectomy (avoiding bile duct injuries)

When in doubt, don't.
Benjamin Franklin

The ultimate goal of any surgeon is to do their operation as safely as possible. Laparoscopic cholecystectomy is one of the basic operations that all general surgeons must perform to be called a real general surgeon. The anatomic proximity of the gallbladder to the bile duct is the essence of the problem. "Stay on the gallbladder wall" is great advice for all gallbladder surgeons but unfortunately the reality is more complicated. Some understanding of the structures adjacent to the wall, porta hepatis and liver, is important for safety. While historically, general surgeons had this knowledge, this ship has now sailed as they no longer operate outside of doing a cholecystectomy. This is a shame, as most general surgeons' anatomic understanding is now confined to just the gallbladder area.

Because of a fatty fibroconnective cover, most of the anatomic structures of the hepatobiliary triangle and porta hepatis go largely unseen (a virtual black box). We all have a very strong bias to only pay attention to what we can immediately see and ignore that which is hidden. Also, the magnification of the laparoscope focuses a surgeon's attention to the very confined area of the upper hepatobiliary triangle. This narrow focus and lack of general anatomic knowledge increases the possibility of a navigational error. The surgeon can become spatially disoriented, effectively lost in space. Unfortunately, the bile duct may be in that space.

Wisdom

A bile duct injury is caused by a navigational error.

Entry problems

The entry into the abdomen with Hassan port placement should be mentioned in every talk on safe cholecystectomy. Disasters await even the most experienced surgeon. The aorta and iliac vessels are immediately below the umbilicus. The brim of the pelvis pushes these vessels forward and in a thin individual they are right there! Damage on entry is 'dead easy'. Further, because this area is not in the laparoscopic field of view, it may go unrecognized until the patient has become unstable from bleeding. Every year patients die from this injury. Bowel injuries are also very common and go largely unreported. The unsuspected cirrhotic patient may have large, high-flow varices around the umbilicus that can lead to significant hemorrhage.

Wisdom

Placing the Hassan trocar can kill.

To steer away from these problems, enter the abdomen by gently tearing open the peritoneum with a finger and stay away from sharp metal instruments. This is done under direct vision. It is even more important when there has been a previous midline incision. Bowel and adhesions can be gently swept away with the same finger. Once a pocket is made, another port can be placed under direct vision. With patience, the upper abdomen can often be safely cleared of significant upper abdominal adhesions. It is important to remember that a blunt finger can still damage bowel. Have a second retrograde look at this area through an upper port before closing.

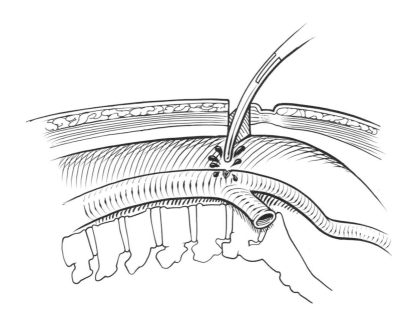

Gallbladder surgery mechanics

To be an expert cholecystectomist, you must have good mechanics. The gallbladder and attached liver must be rotated up from their position covering the duodenum/pancreas. The gallbladder needs to be initially grasped at a level that allows it to be elevated enough to visualize the hepatobiliary triangle. This may require the grasper to be placed well below the fundus. To open the triangle, this grasper also needs to be retracted to the 10 o'clock position. Surgical assistants tend to push the fundus over the top of the triangle to the 2 o'clock position which closes the triangle. The second grasper needs to retract the lower gallbladder/Hartmann's pouch down and lateral towards the appendix! These opposing tensions will give the best view of the hepatobiliary triangle. Lack of a good view can be corrected by increasing the upright position of the patient, releasing Hartmann's pouch from inferior attachments or even placing an additional port for a retracting instrument.

Properly tensioned tissue planes will fall apart when touched with electrocautery. Charring happens when tension is inadequate. Unfortunately, this is often the case in the hepatobiliary triangle; hence, the need for hook cautery. This should always be done on the dissection surface where it can be seen; hooking deep invisible tissue is dangerous. It should be remembered that cauterizing hooked tissue creates a significant collateral burn. The sucker is an excellent blunt tool for finding planes in an inflamed triangle. It also allows the surgeon to do continuous housekeeping, suctioning blood to keep the anatomy clear. The sucker can also be placed in the crotch of the gallbladder and cystic duct to 'tensionize' the triangle. It can also be used to elevate a low Hartmann's pouch and expose the posterior triangle.

The hepatobiliary triangle

All general surgery residents are taught the critical view of safety. This is the clearing of all tissue in the triangle and lower gallbladder plate until only two structures remain (cystic duct and artery). This is an important move and stresses wide exposure and clear identification of structures within the hepatobiliary triangle before any division of tubular structures. It is a form of time-out that arises from the hard won knowledge that the tubular structure at the bottom of the gallbladder is not always the cystic duct. This 'infundibulum' can be the common bile duct fused to the gallbladder, hence narrowing one's attention to the solitary dissection of this area (infundibular technique) is highly risky.

Many surgeons do not understand that by clearing the tissues out of the hepatobiliary triangle the cystic duct is 'unfolded'; this also improves safety by taking the gallbladder away from the bile duct. The right hepatic artery often sits, unrecognized, in the lower triangle. Look for it!

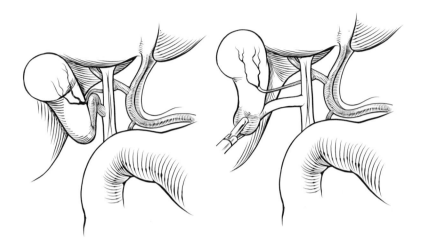

The principles of safe navigation are to move from known areas or landmarks to the unknown. The more landmarks, the safer the movement. That surgeons navigate the operative field is an underappreciated fact. Surgical teachers intuitively use landmarks in every operation but rarely pass these subconscious tips on to their trainees. Because of its proximity to the bile duct, navigation around the gallbladder is crucial. The first landmarks noted by a surgeon are the liver and then the fundus of the gallbladder which immediately orients the surgeon.

Elevation of the gallbladder exposes the subhepatic region and at this point the goal of navigation is to avoid the bile duct. Using the lower part of the gallbladder to navigate is a hazard for two reasons. Inflammation can obliterate the hepatobiliary triangle bringing the gallbladder wall and the bile duct together. The second reason is that the gallbladder may be anatomically situated directly over the bile duct. Clearly, the bottom of the gallbladder is not a good landmark for bile duct avoidance. The cystic duct lymph node is also a poor landmark as inflammatory hypertrophy may place it over the bile duct.

 Wisdom

The bottom of the gallbladder is a poor landmark.

How a 'classic' bile duct injury happens

Understanding how a bile duct injury occurs is important safety knowledge. Making a critical view of safety is a good strategy when anatomy is clear but breaks down when it is not. The hepatobiliary triangle may not exist when the gallbladder is inflamed. For a surgeon who is not familiar with the porta hepatis, it is possible to make a critical view of safety in the porta hepatis, on the left side of the bile duct, instead of the hepatobiliary triangle. This is how a classic bile duct injury occurs.

The surgeon's attention is drawn into the central porta hepatis, on the left side of the bile duct, because of gallbladder inflammation or unusual anatomy. An optical illusion from traction on Hartmann's pouch may kink the bile duct to create a triangle in the central porta hepatis that looks like the hepatobiliary triangle. The common bile duct looks like the cystic duct and the left side of the common hepatic duct looks like the gallbladder wall on top of the triangle.

Wisdom

Any operating on the left side of the bile duct is a 'near miss'.

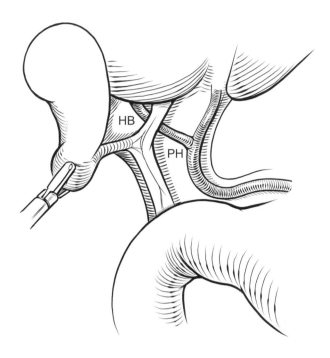

When we operate, we use stored mental images to understand the operative site. We overlay our 'cognitive map' on the area by using key landmarks. This allows us to make a number of assumptions and move the operation forward quickly. When a surgeon, by mistake, places their cholecystectomy cognitive map on the central porta hepatis area, instead of the hepatobiliary triangle, these assumptions are all wrong.

➢ Wisdom

A misplaced 'cognitive map' is the mechanism of classic bile duct injuries.

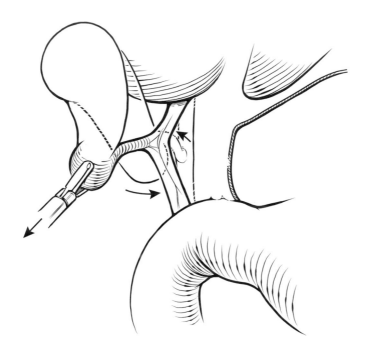

The misplaced map is too far to the left and inferior. The cystic duct part of the map is placed on the common bile duct. This duct is then misinterpreted, clipped and divided. The left side of the common hepatic duct is then dissected as if it were the gallbladder wall and then severed with hook cautery as the surgeon attempts to follow his/her map onto the gallbladder plate. A normal common hepatic duct can be extremely small. It is such a convincing illusion that once the surgeon has entered the correct space under the gallbladder plate, the operation is often completed without recognizing the injury. A piece of duct has been removed; the open common hepatic duct may temporarily seal and not leak bile.

During this process, a critical view of safety may be enlarged on the left side of the bile duct (the portal vein is not recognized) and prosecuted through the hilar plate. The right hepatic artery is often interpreted as a large cystic artery and divided. Bleeding from this artery may be part of the mistake process as bleeding may obscure anatomic landmarks. The basic mistake is that the surgeon has done his dissection too far left and too inferior.

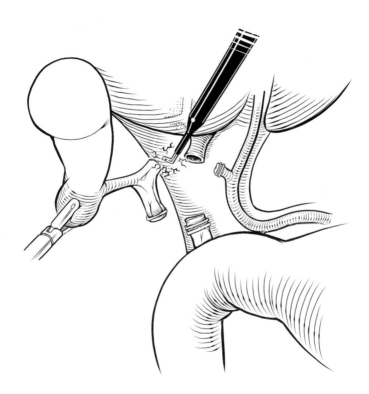

The cognitive triad framework for understanding bile duct injuries

We can now put together a cognitive understanding of how a bile duct injury occurs. There is a triad of basic errors in the surgeon's thought process. These three basic cognitive aspects are: 1) the modern general surgeon's mind; 2) failure of perception (navigation); and 3) failure of correction.

Modern general surgeons now have limited knowledge of the largely invisible porta hepatis anatomy. The framework of a surgeon's dissection does not extend beyond the gallbladder. In other words, their cognitive map is truncated to include only the gallbladder. A lack of open surgery experience in the right upper quadrant (open cholecystectomy and common bile duct exploration) is responsible for this lack of understanding of the entire anatomic field including the liver and duodenum. This is a critical problem as the gallbladder can be in or around the structures of the porta hepatis, most often the bile duct. Further, the laparoscope and its magnification produce the disadvantage of a narrow field of view, reducing landmarks and increasing the risk of navigational errors.

The failure of surgeon perception that occurs in bile duct injuries is not just a simple misinterpretation of anatomy. As discussed, it is a major navigational error with the placement of the surgeon's cognitive map in the wrong location. The starting position is key to playing the piano and surgery; if the piano player does not place her hands in the correct position related to middle C, the following activity does not result in music. The surgeon's instruments in the wrong starting position is equally unpleasant.

Failure of correction of this navigational error occurs for a number of reasons. The piano gives immediate feedback to mispositioned hands, but the surgical field may not. Indeed, the kinked bile duct optical illusion creates an angle in the porta hepatis that mimics the angle in the hepatobiliary area. Our cognitive biases may then take over and keep us on the wrong track. Action bias is the propensity of surgeons to do something and shortcut deeper evaluation of the subhepatic anatomy. Availability bias describes an inability to think of alternate paths of action such as a subtotal cholecystectomy. Confirmation bias is a surgeon's tendency towards cognitive fixation and plan continuation despite contrary evidence such as the unusual proximity of the duodenum to the dissection. Overconfidence and ultimately hubris may explain why these injuries can occur by the hand of a very experienced operator.

A deeper understanding of how surgeons think condensed into a 'cognitive triad' of causes may allow us to develop new strategies to prevent this injury.

 Wisdom

The 'cognitive triad' more deeply explains bile duct injuries.

Avoiding a bile duct injury (navigating away from disaster)

To avoid this soul-destroying nightmare, general surgeons and their residents must be instructed on how to navigate the subhepatic space and porta hepatis by consciously expanding their cognitive maps. Landmarks are the key to safe navigation in any environment. A good surgical landmark must be present often, easy to recognize and give translational information about position (i.e., proximity to the bile duct).

We have studied the cholecystectomy landmarks and found several that meet these criteria. We have named them the five B-SAFE landmarks:

- B stands for bile duct and in at least 70% of patients a portion of it can be seen. Reflecting the duodenum down can demonstrate the duct very effectively.
- S is for the sulcus of Rouvière, a well-established landmark that should always be below the area of dissection.
- A is for the hepatic artery on the left side of the porta. While we cannot see it directly, with a few seconds of concentration we can pick up its pulsation.

- F is for the umbilical fissure that can be seen in almost all patients even when a bridge of liver tissue partly covers it.
- E stand for enteric, the duodenum, which is again universally visible.

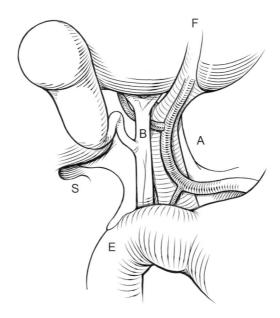

If a surgeon is dissecting within the porta hepatis (too far left and inferior), and checks these landmarks, they will note that they are below the sulcus and too close to the duodenum and too close to the left hepatic artery. A glance up shows they are under the umbilical fissure.

One or two of these landmarks are almost always present, even in an inflamed gallbladder. We suggest they be used in a B-SAFE time-out to be taken before starting the triangle dissection or before cutting the cystic duct. A few seconds to back the camera up and identify the location of the dissection in space with these five landmarks may prevent bile duct mayhem. While this is clearly an 'add-on' strategy to the critical view of safety, it is important to note that the critical view of safety is a strategy that instructs the surgeon on 'where to be'. The B-SAFE time-out instructs the surgeon on 'where NOT to be'.

Wisdom

B-SAFE.

The other point to be made is the danger that hook cautery poses to the bile duct. For some reason, many surgeons, and by default residents, have developed the bad habit of performing the hepatobiliary triangle dissection by placing the hook deep in a hole, turning it on and burning the tissue it catches on the way out — shudder! Not only can this cause an injury to the bile duct side wall or right hepatic artery, it is the mechanism for the upper division of the common hepatic duct in a classic bile duct injury. Nobody does this in open surgery and there is no reason to do it laparoscopically; cautery should be used where you can see it. The other important point for learners is that the dissection is on top of the triangle, on the 'shore' next to the gallbladder wall and not off in the 'sea' of the hepatobiliary triangle.

 Wisdom

Hook cautery is the 'weapon of destruction' for the bile duct.

Sectoral duct injury

Right sectoral ducts are another area of confusion. The anatomy of the bile ducts to the right liver are a wonderful array of inconsistency. Only half of humans have classic anatomy with a single right and left hepatic duct. On the right side there may be separate sectoral ducts. The right posterior sectoral duct can arise from the common hepatic duct (6%) or from a trifurcation or from the left duct. The right anterior sectoral duct can also have an extrahepatic origin from the common duct (18%).

For surgeons operating on the porta hepatis, this means that in about a quarter of cases you will encounter a low riding sectoral duct to the right liver. These sectoral ducts can run closely parallel to the cystic duct or connect directly. They are always at risk of injury. Here, instead of the common bile duct, the sectoral duct is clipped and divided distally and cauterized proximally. The results are different from a classic bile duct injury. The main duct continues to drain normally and the now excluded sectoral duct creates a biloma; after drainage it becomes a biliary fistula. To the casual eye, the ERCP looks 'normal'. Careful scrutiny however, shows a whole area of the liver where the sectoral ductal 'branching tree' is missing. The drain fistulogram or MRCP confirms a large excluded duct that corresponds to the disconnected sector (anterior or posterior) of the liver.

➢ Wisdom

Knowing the anatomy of sectoral duct injuries will amaze your ERCP friends.

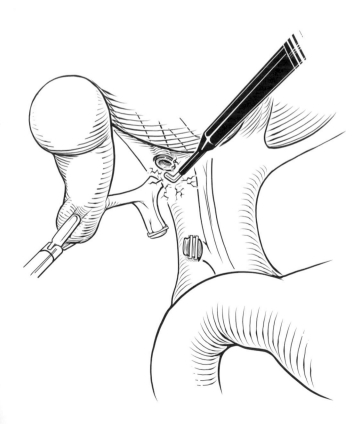

If you are in the operating room shortly after a sectoral duct injury, it is reasonable to do a reconstruction. Otherwise, watchful waiting is the best approach as these excluded duct fistulas will dry up and the affected area of liver will atrophy. As mentioned, do not attempt a delayed hepaticojejunostomy as these damaged ducts are very small and encased in fibrous inflammatory tissue. Remote reconstruction has a high failure rate. A chronic poorly-vascularized liver sector with cholangitis can be resected down the road. You may be consulted on a patient with right sectoral liver atrophy with dilated ducts remote from a laparoscopic cholecystectomy. They have had an unrecognized sectoral duct injury at their original gallbladder surgery. If they are asymptomatic leave them alone.

In spite of the literature describing posterior sectoral duct injury, a right anterior duct injury is significantly more common.

Wisdoms

- *A bile duct injury is caused by a navigational error.*

- *Placing the Hassan trocar can kill.*

- *The bottom of the gallbladder is a poor landmark.*

- *Any operating on the left side of the bile duct is a 'near miss'.*

- *A misplaced 'cognitive map' is the mechanism of classic bile duct injuries.*

- *The 'cognitive triad' more deeply explains bile duct injuries.*

- *B-SAFE.*

- *Hook cautery is the 'weapon of destruction' for the bile duct.*

- *Knowing the anatomy of sectoral duct injuries will amaze your ERCP friends.*

Chapter 19

The difficult cholecystectomy

It's not what you look at that matters, it's what you see.
Henry David Thoreau

Part of being an HPB surgeon is operating on difficult gallbladders. The morbidly obese patient, the cirrhotic patient, and the comorbid patient are all yours. It is important to remember that just because you are the 'expert' does not mean that all these gallbladders have to be removed. Patients are always asking to just have their stones removed. This is rarely done as, of course, there is no surgical billing code for stone removal. However, they actually have a point. We can have the interventional radiologist place a percutaneous drain in the gallbladder and then with upsizing and a little effort, fish out all the offending stones. It works and can save a patient with advanced cholecystitis and a heart that does not pump from a regrettable operation.

If you do find yourself in the operating room with a 'cholecystitis bomb', you need a strategy. Because you are expert, you can push the operation safely beyond just placing a drain and save patients multiple reinterventions. The key here is to be patient and work your way onto the gallbladder wall. You need to stay there as you work your way down, until your 'spider senses' start to tingle. In other words, your B-SAFE landmarks are telling you that you have strayed into the porta hepatis and bile duct territory (too far left and inferior). Don't expect there to be a hepatobiliary triangle. At this point you need to back-up the gallbladder to a known area. This area, if it exists, is back on the liver-gallbladder interface. Create a window here between the gallbladder and liver. This may orient you enough to make some further dissection inferiorly. At some undefined point you need to chicken out and open the gallbladder and take out the stones. We place a retrieval bag below the gallbladder to catch the stones and debris as we work. A little look inside may also allow further dissection. You can then remove the upper gallbladder and any remaining stones. The stump can be closed with an endoloop or sutures. Getting out the endostapler should be avoided. Inability to close the stump is not a tragedy as a drain will result in a controlled fistula if the cystic duct is still open. This fistula will usually close without bile duct instrumentation. Congratulations, you have just done a subtotal cholecystectomy.

➢ Wisdom

When in trouble think 'subtotal'.

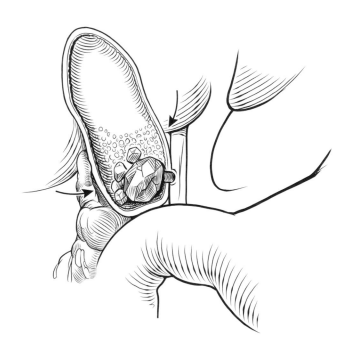

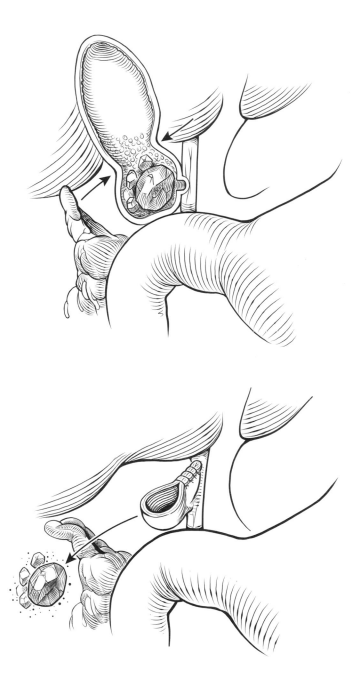

It is important to have a strong understanding of the 'inflammatory peel' that often forms around an inflamed gallbladder. This thick rind of inflammatory tissue offers a path around the gallbladder. There are hazards though. You must pay attention to what layer of the peel you are dissecting. Better to be closer to the gallbladder mucosa as duodenum and bile duct can make up part of the wall. If the peel does not come away easily, stop before you start making holes.

On a technical note, much of the gallbladder dissection can be done bluntly. The surgical sucker is a tool that will develop planes and remove blood and other fluid at the same time. Trainees need to watch and practice using this instrument. Digging out an inflamed Hartmann's pouch can be a defining move.

➤ Wisdom

The sucker is the tool of choice for the difficult gallbladder.

Wisdoms

- *When in trouble think 'subtotal'.*

- *The sucker is the tool of choice for the difficult gallbladder.*

Chapter 20

Bile duct injury repair

It's not what happens to you, but how you react to it that matters.

Epictetus

Early bile duct injury repair

The best thing for the patient and the equally traumatized surgeon is to repair a bile duct injury with a Roux-en-Y hepaticojejunostomy immediately after it has happened. The results of an immediately recognized bile duct injury with intraoperative HPB surgical repair is excellent. Conversion to open surgery is necessary to gain wide exposure.

Once you have established there has been a major injury it is probably best to open and get all your tools. Then a meticulous dissection should allow definition of all the anatomic structures of the porta hepatis and hepatobiliary triangle. An injured right hepatic artery, that cannot be easily repaired, should be tied off. There is an excellent collateral blood supply to the right bile ducts and common hepatic duct through the left hepatic artery via a hilar plate blood vessel network. In a major injury you are often looking directly at the portal vein. Any portal vein injury should be repaired with fine sutures. If the duct is completely transected, a hepaticojejunostomy is required. Side wall injuries can be sutured or in rare circumstances be repaired over a T-tube.

Reconstruction can be difficult. Like operating on a pediatric bile duct, it is surprising how small and thin-walled a normal bile duct can be. In the rare event of a clean (non-cautery) cut, it is possible to sew the ends back together. A hepaticojejunostomy is usually a better idea. The bile duct anastomosis should not be done to the severed end of the bile duct as the cautery injury can make the end of this duct suspect. It is important to cut the duct back closer to the level of the hilar plate (duct bleeding here is a good sign). If there is an injury to a sectoral duct it should also be clearly identified and cut back towards the plate before reconstruction. Magnification may be necessary to connect small ducts to the Roux limb with fine sutures. Going very high above the bifurcation and through the hilar plate (Hepp-Couinaud repair) in these early reconstructions is usually not necessary.

If the patient is not referred immediately, most HPB surgeons will still reoperate up to a week after the injury, as long as the patient is stable and not septic. The timing of reoperation is not well defined but doing a connection in a severely inflamed porta hepatis is to be avoided.

Postoperatively, full disclosure to the patient and family should be provided by both surgeons. While this may not necessarily prevent legal action, it is just the right thing to do. Careful documentation of the events in an immediately dictated operative report should be done by the staff surgeon and not a resident or fellow. The original operating surgeon should be encouraged to do likewise.

 Wisdom

Immediate repair of a bile duct injury is best.

If the patient presents or is transferred late from the injury with bile in the peritoneal cavity and sepsis, you are now in the business of saving their life and not repairing the duct. Resuscitation, antibiotics, ICU support and getting the leak drained properly are the agenda items. A laparotomy or laparoscopic washout may be necessary. Percutaneous transhepatic drains may be useful but are often not necessary. An ERCP may be useful in diagnosing and stenting a cystic duct stump leak.

Remote bile duct injury repair

When the duct is not repaired immediately it is probably best to wait several months. This gives time for the inflammation to subside and the complete anatomy to be delineated. MRI, CT, CT angiogram and cholangiograms through the drains can give a clear picture. The wait will also allow the duct to be repaired to dilate and thicken.

At surgery, expect it to be scarred and difficult. Following the drain can be a good strategy to get you to the bile duct. It is also important to remember the hilar plate and the left bile duct are there for your pleasure. The proximal left duct can be opened for a wide anastomosis. If the duct cannot be delineated from below the bifurcation, lower the hilar plate and access the left hepatic duct through the plate (Hepp-Couinaud repair). This jargon is somewhat confusing. What is really meant here is that, in a high injury, you have to get into the liver to get a good connection. This can mean a number of things. The left hepatic duct can be accessed by dissecting segment 4b off the hilar plate and finding the left hepatic duct running within the plate (use a needle probe if necessary).

➢ Wisdom

Exposure of the hilar plate is the window for delayed bile duct repair.

Anomalies of the left hepatic duct are frequent. Thirty-five percent of patients will have two left hepatic ducts within the hilar plate. These are still amenable to bypass and can be connected for a single anastomosis.

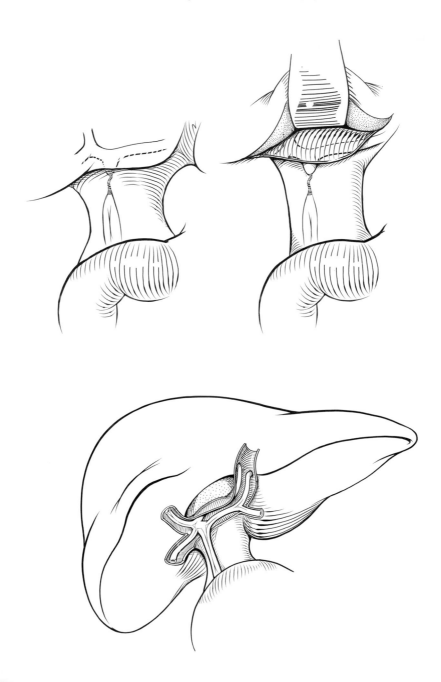

A high injury may require segmental liver resection above the porta hepatis on either the right or left sides. The right ducts are always harder to access as they drop back into the liver quickly and are more likely to require some liver parenchyma removal to expose them clearly. As mentioned, an isolated injury to the right sectoral duct should only be operated on if the patient is symptomatic (prolonged fistula or cholangitis). This mandates a right liver resection rather than bile duct reconstruction. Delayed hepaticojejunostomy to a right sectoral duct is notoriously difficult due to their size and surrounding scar tissue. As a result, they typically lead to long-term strictures and ongoing cholangitis requiring eventual resection anyway.

 Wisdom

Don't be shy; resect liver to expose a high duct for repair.

Patients that develop late strictures from duct injuries presenting with recurrent cholangitis are usually not jaundiced. A trial of stenting may obviate reconstructive surgery even if it has a lower overall success rate.

All of these patients need to be followed with serial yearly liver function tests as late strictures can occur.

Hilar plate injuries

Injuries through the hilar plate require special consideration. The basic mechanism of this injury is the same as the classic bile duct injury taken to the extreme. Instead of just cauterizing through the common hepatic duct, the disoriented surgeon takes the dissection through the hilar plate and left hepatic duct(s), pulls the plate down and then divides the right side of the plate extending into the origin of the right anterior and posterior sectoral bile ducts. The bile duct bifurcation with hilar plate is removed and depending on variations in anatomy this can leave 2-5 small bile ducts for reconstruction. Caudate ducts are too small to repair and should be sutured if they are found.

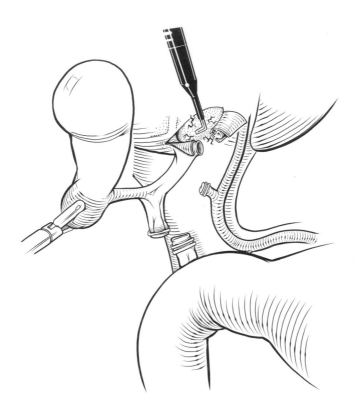

It is important to recognize that the collateral blood supply to the right liver/bile duct has been removed. If the right hepatic artery proper is also gone and there is no non-regressed right hepatic artery, the bile ducts in the right liver are permanently devascularized. Connections to these ducts leak, stricture and eventually result in a chronically infected (cholangitis) shrunken area of liver. If this situation is recognized in an early repair, this is the one circumstance where right hepatic artery reconstruction is reasonable. Surgeons doing a late repair to a known dearterialized right liver should consider resection. The problem is that the extent of the plate injury may not be appreciated prior to the exploration. Practically, a right duct connection may have to be made and liver resection held in reserve. The patient may then develop chronic cholangitis and show a clear indication for a right hepatectomy. Rarely, a severe central hilar plate injury may require liver transplantation after secondary biliary cirrhosis develops.

Help in the gallbladder operating room

Rather than just repairing damaged bile ducts, helping prevent the injury in the first place is a laudable goal. Many HPB surgery services offer a kind of informal 'flying advice program' for general surgeons struggling with difficult cholecystectomies. This may involve simple telephone advice all the way up to attending the surgery and repairing a severed duct. Your availability and willingness to help, in a non-critical way, is an important part of safe surgery in your institution. If young surgeons are too afraid to call, you have a real problem.

It is incumbent on you to train young residents and general surgeons to do a safe subtotal cholecystectomy and in hard cases (when you cannot get there) to drain and get out. Surgeons should be discouraged from doing 3-hour laparoscopic cholecystectomies. When you are there, nothing is wrong with teaching the art of navigation with the utilization of landmarks. When it is a question of duct injury, your immediate attendance is optimal. Beware the phone call where a small accessory duct has been found; it is often a transected hepatic duct. Out of town patients should be drained, transported and operated on, as soon as possible.

➤ Wisdom

A leaking accessory duct is often a severed common hepatic duct.

The first thing to do on entering anyone else's operating room is to be respectful. You are there to help not to criticize. Determine the stability of the patient and obtain the quick facts. Rather than immediately delving into the operation, orient the operative field. What are the structures and where is the surgeon operating (do a B-SAFE time-out)? Often a little reorientation will get the surgeon out of the wrong spot (left side of the bile duct) and allow the operation to proceed. You do not necessarily have to take over. If there is significant bleeding it may be best to open and control (remember your Pringle). Bile coming from 'where it should not' is also a reason to convert to open surgery.

If any type of repair is necessary, it is probably best to take over the patient's postoperative care. Keep the original surgeon informed and encourage them to visit and follow-up on their patient. Use your words carefully so as to not cast medicolegal aspersions. You will likely find yourself in this same situation at some point in your career. A little hand holding and soft supportive banter will also help.

Bile duct injuries can produce a whole spectrum of denial and other types of surgeon misbehavior (sending the patient to a gastroenterologist, etc.). It is important to note that HPB surgeons do not injure bile ducts but instead do en bloc resections of gallbladder/bile duct masses suspicious for cancer!

➢ Wisdom

A surgeon who has cut a bile duct (or is about to) needs all aspects of your support.

Wisdoms

- *Immediate repair of a bile duct injury is best.*

- *Exposure of the hilar plate is the window for delayed bile duct repair.*

- *Don't be shy; resect liver to expose a high duct for repair.*

- *A leaking accessory duct is often a severed common hepatic duct.*

- *A surgeon who has cut a bile duct (or is about to) needs all aspects of your support.*

Chapter 21

Gallbladder special circumstances

Excellence is a habit.
Aristotle

Cholecystectomy in morbidly obese patients

All your tricks need to be pulled out when removing a gallbladder in a morbidly obese patient. It is important to have a plan and extra-long ports. Strap the patient to the OR table so you can get them upright. Gravity has to work for you. The Hassan port should be placed significantly above the umbilicus to allow vision over the omentum. Be sure the ports are angled correctly so you don't have to spend an hour of hard torquing on the abdominal wall. A fatty liver will limit gallbladder retraction so extra ports for retraction may be necessary. The fatty liver may also push into the hepatobiliary triangle making for a contracted space that is awkward to dissect. These can be highly morbid procedures. Talk to the patient and remember percutaneous drainage and stone removal are an option. An open conversion is likely to be equally difficult and morbid for the patient.

Open cholecystectomy

The whole issue of converting to an open procedure is at your discretion. You are now part of a rare breed, a surgeon comfortable performing an open cholecystectomy. For the new generation of general surgeons, an open operation may not offer an advantage over the laparoscopic approach. They will call you, or drain the gallbladder and then send the patient to you later.

If you do open, the principles are the same, take out as much of the gallbladder as is safe and don't forget to take out all the stones. It is perhaps easier in open surgery, to maintain a cuff of gallbladder wall and close the stump with interrupted sutures (subtotal cholecystectomy).

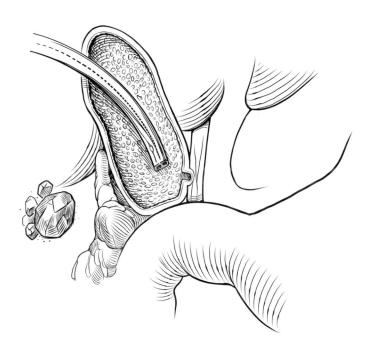

Most patients with a part of their gallbladder left inside never have issues. However, failure to remove all the stones may result in recurrent cholecystitis and a nasty reoperation to remove the inflamed gallbladder stump. Hemicholecystectomy is OK as long as you remove the stones. In particularly bad gallbladders, all you may be able to get out is a small patch of anterior gallbladder wall. No problem, stones out and then drain in.

➢ Wisdom

It's the stones, silly! Take out the stones.

Useful tricks for open cholecystectomy are the same as for liver surgery. Use your two-posted retractor and obtain wide exposure. Often the gallbladder is deep in the right upper quadrant. Bringing it down and to the left can be accomplished by placing packs. The packs need to go above the dome and to the side of segment 6. It is surprising how readily this brings the gallbladder into an operable space under the incision. Above and below retractor blades will expose a difficult hepatobiliary triangle by pulling up on liver segment 4 and down on the bowel. It is unlikely you will have an experienced assistant to help you do this.

If you are doing a primary open cholecystectomy in a hostile abdomen, make the incision right over the gallbladder fundus (subcostal). Your CT scan or drain site will show you where this is. This direct approach avoids the potential for collateral damage from long dissection from a distant midline incision.

Stones in the bile duct

The fun that surgeons used to have removing stones from the common bile duct is now over. Old surgeons remember the common trainee question: what are the indications for exploring the common duct? If you ask that question now, you will receive a bewildered stare. Of course, the modern answer is: when ERCP has failed; and this is not very often. Endoscopists will repeat this procedure for weeks before giving up with 'ERCP fatigue syndrome'. Only then will the patient be passed on to the HPB surgeon. Rarely, an ERCP stone basket can irreversibly ensnare an unretrievable stone and require immediate common duct exploration.

There is an increasing volume of patients in our communities who have had Roux-en-Y gastric bypass procedures for morbid obesity. Common duct stones in these patients require some thought. Success with balloon endoscopic ERCP is reported, but requires a skilled and motivated endoscopist. Interventional radiologists are also now equipped to remove moderately sized common duct stones with a transhepatic approach. Whether this is less risk than an open operation remains to be confirmed. Recently, there has been considerably less noise about laparoscopic common duct exploration. If you are experienced in this procedure it is perhaps a reasonable application. To us, it makes no sense to perform a laparoscopic duct exploration if the common duct is accessible endoscopically. Manipulating or cutting open a small-calibre duct should be avoided as there is always a risk of postoperative bile leakage or late stricture formation. At the end of the day, this leaves too few patients to maintain broad-based surgical expertise with the laparoscopic approach. However, there is still room for creativity here: doing the laparoscopic cholecystectomy in a combined surgical interventional radiology suite or giving the 'ERCPist' surgical access through the stomach with a temporary gastrostomy.

Before you jump at a common bile duct exploration, be sure of two things: first, that the stones are actually causing problems and second, that your patient will survive the operation. Asymptomatic patients with small stones can be given a trial of observations as most will pass without problems. If they have ongoing pain or partial obstruction, find an old surgical atlas and go for it. Open the duct vertically and use stay sutures to keep it open if needed. Use irrigation and Fogarty® catheters to avoid impacting stones into the ampulla. Use the choledochoscope and stone forceps out of the hospital catacombs. If the senior surgeon helping out pulls out the Bakes dilators, put them away quickly. Sew up the bile duct with 5.0 polydioxanone (PDS®) or smaller sutures and try to avoid a T-tube. Nobody on the surgical ward knows how to take care of these things anymore. If the duct leaks have your friend in the ERCP suite place an endoscopic bile duct stent.

➤ Wisdom

Avoid T-tubes; nobody knows what they are anymore.

Only if the duct is inaccessible to ERCP or you are reconstructing a partially damaged duct (Mirizzi syndrome) is a T-tube a good idea. If you are forced into this there are several principles to follow. Make the limbs short and cut out part of the back wall adjacent to the T to allow easy removal. Secure the tube at the abdominal wall with a little slack so when the patient stretches or twists, the T-tube does not pop out of the bile duct. The direction from duct to the abdominal wall should be relatively straight. Get a T-tube cholangiogram prior to removal to assure the duct is clear. A fibrous tract will form in about a week but it is judicious to wait at least 3 weeks before removal, longer if the patient is immunosuppressed. Warn the patient it may leak a little bile for the first 12 hours.

A transduodenal sphincteroplasty is an even more rare event; an impacted stone and no access via ERCP remains the indication. Get the duodenum fully mobilized by Kocherization, and make a small antimesenteric duodenotomy directly over the palpable stone. Find the ampulla with gentle palpation, cannulate and open it slightly off vertically to the patient's right (11 o'clock) to avoid the orifice of the pancreatic duct. The 'plasty' is actually a side-to-side anastomosis from the duodenal wall to the common bile duct. It must be done with fine sutures; a cannula in the pancreatic duct can be used to landmark and help orient away from this orifice.

Intraoperative cholangiogram

The issue of performing an intraoperative cholangiogram at the time of cholecystectomy has taken on aspects of a religious mantra in many places. While having the 'tools' to do a cholangiogram is useful, cutting a hole in an unknown duct and then placing and securing a cholangiogram catheter is perhaps not the best way to find the main bile duct. You may create the duct injury you are trying to avoid. Also, routine operative cholangiography will inevitably find some small duct stones and doing ERCP intervention in these patients may be worse than the disease. Most will pass with an innocuous burp. Further, most surgeons are just too lazy to do what is a 20-minute fiddle to obtain an X-ray that they are no longer competent to interpret. The time for routine intraoperative cholangiography has therefore passed. Other new options exist that offer less invasive advantages, including routine laparoscopic ultrasound of the common duct or indocyanine green fluorescent cholangiography.

Gallbladder plate injury

This is the plate you want to stay under (not like the hilar or umbilical plate) when performing laparoscopic cholecystectomies. It contains structures that are best avoided. Bile ducts in the plate, or just under it, have variously been called ducts of Luschka and have been responsible for generations of confusion. They are not cholecystohepatic ducts (ducts connecting to the gallbladder), which are extremely rare. In any case, if you invade the plate and cut a duct of Luschka, they can leak. This most often causes a little postoperative discomfort before they self-seal. Occasionally though, it's the full monty with a bile collection, requiring drainage and bile duct decompression with ERCP stenting. Better not to go there and leave the plate intact.

The other reason to respect the plate is that the superficial branch of the middle hepatic vein hides just under it in about 30% of patients. It is always a nasty bleeding surprise to get into this vein. Pressure with a forceps gauze is a good first step. A good cautery created eschar plug can usually get you out of this bind and seal the bleeding vein. Applying the strategy of hemorrhage control learned from laparoscopic liver resections may be necessary. Uncontrolled bleeding may occasionally require open conversion and suturing. Rarely, a small artery can also be found within the plate.

 Wisdom

Respect the gallbladder plate.

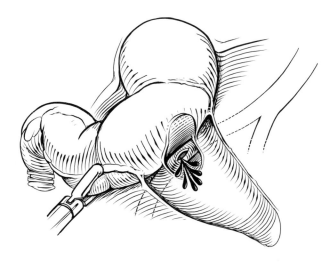

Mirizzi syndrome

'Mirizzi' — what a wonderful name. It sounds like chaos and that is not far from the truth. The crux of the problem is an impacted gallstone at the bottom of the gallbladder that pushes into the cystic duct and then erodes into the common bile duct. The cystic duct eventually ceases to exist. This process creates tremendous local inflammation in what is a critical area. It may or may not produce jaundice but it always results in a confused ERCPist. A pathopneumonic presentation is a referral from your endoscopist where there is biliary obstruction and a common duct stone that cannot be removed. The stone is impacted and may still have a rim of remaining cystic duct holding it from basket removal.

An MR cholangiogram will often show a stone in a dilated distal cystic duct that has pushed into the common bile duct. How long this has been going on determines how much of the bile duct is destroyed. It is a slight misnomer to call this a simple fistula creation. Occasionally, a very large portion of the anterior wall of the bile duct is missing. While it can be formally classified, it is important to remember that this is a continuous process.

➢ Wisdom

Mirizzi syndrome is the 'helter skelter' of biliary surgery.

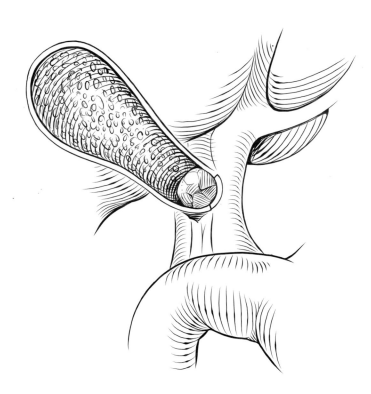

Regardless, the approach is the same. An open approach is probably best but there are some virtuoso laparoscopists that are capable enough to do this. Take the body of the gallbladder out and fish out the stone from inside the gallbladder stump. Avoid a direct attack on the porta hepatis as it is inflamed and full of hazard. The key is getting the stone out and then closing the gallbladder stump with or without a T-tube or stent. In cases where the side of the bile duct is destroyed, the gallbladder stump may be used to effectively reconstruct a new bile duct. Remember to leave a cuff of gallbladder wall at the start so you can reconstruct at the end. While biliary reconstruction with a hepaticojejunostomy may be necessary, it is a default option. The differential diagnosis here is gallbladder cancer. Sometimes it is difficult to delineate the two so always get a piece of tissue for pathology and pay attention to the result.

➢ Wisdom

Leave some gallbladder wall to reconstruct the bile duct.

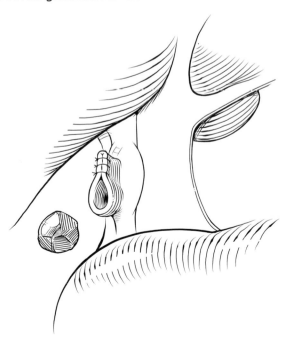

'Erosive' cholecystitis

Mirizzi syndrome is a situation of gallstone erosion into the common bile duct. Remember though that gallstones can erode into any surrounding structure. It is part of a syndrome we have labelled 'erosive cholecystitis'. The other common site is the duodenum. This is because *in situ* the gallbladder often lays adjacent to the duodenal wall. Direct erosion can result in the stone creating a fistula into the duodenum with the stone eventually dropping in for a visit. The decompression of the gallbladder can resolve symptoms of cholecystitis only to be replaced with obstructive symptoms as the gallstone travels down the bowel. It is unclear why this is called gallstone ileus, as no ileus occurs. Gallstones can erode into other locations including stomach or colon or even just into the peritoneal space.

➢ Wisdom

A gallbladder fistula cures cholecystitis without cholecystectomy.

Prolonged inflammation can effectively destroy some, or all, of the gallbladder wall. It is important to know this as efforts to remove something that is departed will only damage surrounding structures, most likely duodenum. Indeed, in most cases of erosive cholecystitis (except Mirizzi syndrome), removal of the gallbladder is not a good idea. Fistula formation and stone drop-out effectively cures the cholecystitis. You do not need to fix the fistula!

➢ Wisdom

Stay on the gallbladder wall.

The gallbladder wall might not exist.

Wisdom

Don't try to take out something that does not exist.

Sump syndrome

Years ago, there was a body of thought that a large dilated common bile duct with many stones should be decompressed into the duodenum. A side-to-side connection was made (choledochoduodenostomy). These patients may be still walking around and even present with pancreatitis or just pain, as the stones and debris collect in the distal common bile duct sump. Imaging may be confusing. An endoscopic sphincterotomy will solve most of these problems but occasionally the duct connection has to be redone with a formal end-to-side hepaticojejunostomy and duodenal wall repair.

Complicated biliary fistula

At some point, a complicated patient with an inflammatory bomb below the liver and multiple biliary fistulae will show you what real misery can be. They often present after a gallbladder surgical misadventure. Resist the urge to offer an immediate surgical cure. Delineate the anatomy, ducts leaking, surrounding bowel and blood vessels that may have been damaged. Doing a contrast X-ray through the drains can often show the complicated biliary anatomy.

 Wisdom

Contrast X-rays through a drain with bile staining is a biliary reality show.

The patient can often be very unwell physically and mentally traumatised. This is a situation to drain, wait, and support, even if it means a prolonged hospital stay. Some of these scenarios are not fixable and you have to palliate a non-cancer patient.

Gallbladder cancer

Tumors of the gallbladder are common. Undiagnosed masses in the gallbladder wall are more common. The surgical treatment of gallbladder cancer revolves around the prevention of bile/tumor spillage. When the gallbladder with a cancer is entered in any way, cure becomes difficult. For this reason, biopsy is not reasonable for a gallbladder mass. Casual removal by an unsuspecting general surgeon is equally bad. Primary wide extended resection of a gallbladder mass is the goal. Herein lies a problem; inflammation and cancer can be indistinguishable. This means that a radical approach is required for all suspicious lesions. If your general surgeon buddy asks you to look at a gallbladder mass intraoperatively, always tell him it could be a cancer and take over. Nobody can definitively diagnose gallbladder cancer with their eyes.

Gallbladder polyps at around 1cm are rarely cancers and polyps greater than 2cm are mostly cancers. It is your public health mandate to remove gallbladders with polyps greater than 1cm.

 Wisdom

A gallbladder with a possible cancer needs to remain intact until it sees the pathologist.

For small fundal lesions we have adopted a laparoscopic approach with dissection of the lower gallbladder including plate and extending to a liver resection higher up around the mass. If cancer in the pathological specimen is confirmed, regional lymph node dissection is reasonable. For all other lesions an open approach is probably best. The goal is to never spill bile. Occasionally, very aggressive surgeries need to be pursued including liver, duodenum and colon resections. Many of these end up being inflammatory on pathology — sigh! The extent of liver resection required remains undefined. The goal is to get a negative margin so several centimeters of non-anatomic parenchyma is reasonable. Perhaps the whole of segments 4b/5 do not need to be removed. Regional portal lymph node dissection will give important prognostic information but is unlikely to improve the cancer-related outcome.

Cancers found on cholecystectomy specimen on pathology should initiate staging and reoperation to remove regional liver and nodes. A history of bile spillage is a marker for poor prognosis. Large tumors invading the porta hepatis and causing jaundice are bad actors and are very difficult to cure. However, it is worth exploring patients with limited porta hepatis involvement. Aggressive combined liver, bile duct and lymph node resection is the only option for these patients. Resection of preceding laparoscopic port sites remains debatable, but reasonable.

Wisdoms

- *It's the stones, silly! Take out the stones.*

- *Avoid T-tubes; nobody knows what they are anymore.*

- *Respect the gallbladder plate.*

- *Mirizzi syndrome is the 'helter skelter' of biliary surgery.*

- *Leave some gallbladder wall to reconstruct the bile duct.*

- *A gallbladder fistula cures cholecystitis without cholecystectomy.*

- *Stay on the gallbladder wall.*

- *The gallbladder wall might not exist.*

- *Don't try to take out something that does not exist.*

- *Contrast X-rays through a drain with bile staining is a biliary reality show.*

- *A gallbladder with a possible cancer needs to remain intact until it sees the pathologist.*

Section V

Pancreas

More than any other organ, operating on the pancreas requires special wisdom. Your mother will forgive you, the pancreas won't. First, it is in an awkward position; in the retroperitoneum behind stomach and colon. It is intimate with the duodenum. Large vessels transgress its integrity. It is soft, friable and responds to disease by becoming hard and adhesed to surrounding structures. There is no mesentery or vascular leash for controlling blood vessels going in or out. Lastly, it contains enzymes that at the slightest transgression can leak and ruin your day. The short answer is that you need a good reason to operate on this organ with a clear and limited set of goals.

Chapter 22

Pancreatic anatomy

Wisdom is the right use of knowledge. To know is not to be wise.
Many men know a great deal, and are all the greater fools for it.
There is no fool so great as a knowing fool.
But to know how to use knowledge is to have wisdom.
Charles Spurgeon

Pancreas orientation

One should think of the pancreas as folding itself over the aorta and vena cava. This means the central pancreas is most anterior and easiest to expose. Both right and especially left sides tend to drift posteriorly into the flanks. This also exposes the pancreas neck and body to blunt abdominal trauma. The duodenal/pancreas complex forms a 'crossroads' of the upper abdomen with bowel, vessels and ducts all interdigitating in a confined area. It is possible to conceptualize this area in four layers. The covering layer is stomach and omentum, colon and mesentery. The money layer is duodenum, pancreas and spleen. The danger layer is the mesenteric/hepatic arteries and portal venous circulation. The base layer is the inferior vena cava, aorta, kidney and adrenals. Pancreatic operations are largely about separating these layers.

> ## ➢ Wisdom

The pancreas/duodenal complex is the 'crossroads' of the abdomen.

Transverse colon mesentery

The mesentery of the transverse colon is a big player in pancreas exposure. It attaches under the body of the pancreas and extends across the head. The mesentery contains many important vessels (middle colic, right colic and origin of the mesenteric veins). To expose the pancreatic head and body this mesentery must be dissected with special attention to these veins. The veins can also be used as landmarks that lead to critical structures (i.e., the right and middle colic veins show the way to the superior mesenteric vein [SMV]; the inferior mesenteric vein [IMV] shows the way to the splenic vein). Mobilizing the mesentery of the colon splenic flexure is key to exposing the tail of the pancreas. Similarly, mobilizing the mesentery to the hepatic flexure of the colon is key to exposing the head of the pancreas.

➤ Wisdom

You have to know the transverse colon mesentery to expose the pancreas.

Splanchnic veins

The portal venous circulation dominates the pancreas. The transit of these veins around and under the pancreas are central to any operation on the pancreas. The pancreas forms around these veins in utero. Small to large venous tributaries are always potential trouble. Tumor encroachment on the portal vein can be the difference between resection and palliation. The vein walls are all essential landmarks, the transit of the superior mesenteric vein (SMV)/portal vein (PV) under the pancreatic neck being the most important. The area on top of the vein typically has no tributaries and allows the creation of a tunnel. There is also significant variability. The splenic vein can connect to the SMV anywhere behind the pancreatic neck. The inferior mesenteric vein may connect anywhere from the mid-splenic to the side of the SMV.

The gastrocolic trunk is the key tributary arising from the right side of the SMV just below the pancreatic neck. It is broad-based, but quickly branches into a right colic and gastroepiploic branches. It should be divided to open the entire window to the tunnel under the neck of the pancreas. The difference between a master pancreatic surgeon and a rookie is often the initial breadth of attack and generous exposure of this area when resecting tumors of the pancreatic neck.

The splenic vein tends to become more encompassed/enveloped by the pancreas as one gets closer to the spleen. Centrally near the SMV it is separate from the pancreas. In its mid position it is in a groove, but in the pancreatic tail, it can interdigitate with pancreas parenchyma as it splits into splenic tributaries. Small short and nasty veins drain the pancreas directly into the splenic vein at variable sites.

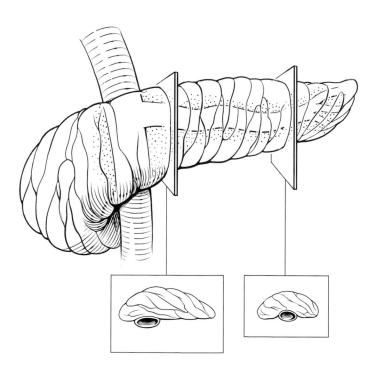

Pancreatic head

The head of the pancreas is a complicated three-dimensional structure. It is nestled around the superior mesenteric vein. It wraps around and dives under the SMV as the uncinate process. In combination with the duodenum, the pancreatic head has a rich arterial blood supply from anastomosing pancreatoduodenal arteries arising from the superior mesenteric (SMA) and hepatic arteries. There is a small fatty mesentery from the distal stomach/duodenum that contains gastroepiploic vessels. This mesentery often overlays the pancreatic head and obscures the more proximal gastroduodenal artery.

The gastroduodenal artery floats over the top edge of the pancreas and onto its surface, to the right of the neck. The SMA remains largely invisible through most pancreatic operations (unless it is dissected out during a pancreatic head resection). It is left and inferior to the SMV but can occasionally loop to the right and expose itself to potential damage by an unsuspecting surgeon. A practiced hand can orient by feeling for the SMA position.

Pancreatic body and tail

The body and tail of the pancreas extend under the stomach with the anterior peritoneal covering of the lesser sac. It can push deep into the splenic hilum. The pancreatic body covers the left adrenal gland which may occasionally create a surprise during posterior dissection. The shape of the pancreatic body may be round or relatively flat and is always somewhat irregular. The splenic artery runs a looping course under and above the top edge of the pancreas. Its course can occasionally surprise with extreme tortuosity. At its origin, the coeliac axis, it can be difficult to find as it is covered with dense nerve and fibrous tissue. As with all vessels, the best dissection plane is right next to the artery wall. Be careful with energy devices, however, as imperceptible collateral burns to the arterial wall are the origins of pseudoaneurysm formation and late postoperative bleeds.

The ducts in the pancreas are relatively consistent. The pancreatic duct tends to be posterior and superior in the body. The common bile duct is medial to the pancreatic duct in the head, in roughly the same plane.

Pancreas duodenal relationship

The duodenum becomes intimate with the pancreatic head following the pylorus. There is usually several centimeters past the pylorus where it can be divided before arriving at the pancreas. The duodenum becomes more retroperitoneal as one moves around the C-loop towards the fourth part. As it goes under the mesenteric vessels, it may extend down as far as the pelvic brim. Just to make life interesting, it can occasionally transit left higher up, directly under the pancreas. It emerges on the left side of the vessels as proximal jejunum with the start of small bowel mesentery. The ligament of Treitz, which is often invisible and posterior to the pancreas, is composed of a fibromuscular suspensory band of tissue that holds the duodenojejunal junction up towards the inferior border of the pancreas. We have yet to actually see this 'ligament', but have it on good authority that it really exists. The evidence is that the proximal jejunum is often pulled into the inferior edge of the pancreas (beware). There is an odd peritoneal depression in this area. The inferior mesenteric vein is often found on the far side of this depression. The SMV and uncinate are close in this area but rarely visible from the left side.

Wisdoms

- *The pancreas/duodenal complex is the 'crossroads' of the abdomen.*

- *You have to know the transverse colon mesentery to expose the pancreas.*

Chapter 23

Pancreatic procedures

Never laugh at live dragons.
J.R.R. Tolkien

Preoperative pancreatic surgery issues

For most patients, high-quality triphasic computed tomography is all that is required to plan pancreatic surgery. High fidelity and appropriately timed venous phase imaging are the key sequences to review. Most HPB surgeons will unconsciously evaluate the SMV/portal vein first. Sagittal reconstruction can be enlightening as it shows the portal superior mesenteric vein in its longitudinal dimension. This is where the money is; it is surprising how often the radiology report does not do this area justice. Useful calcification patterns can be readily identified on CT. Arterial phase images are important to delineate hypervascular versus hypovascular lesions, as well as arterial anatomy. The downside of CT scans remains detection of small liver and peritoneal metastases. MRI and MR cholangiography will offer a better view of liver metastases, ductal anatomy and stones in special circumstances.

Endoscopic ultrasound (EUS) can also be an extremely useful procedure. For small lesions of the distal bile duct and ampulla, EUS findings can be very illuminating. In special circumstances, needle biopsy of pancreatic lesions and or surrounding lymph nodes can reveal a definitive diagnosis and guide treatment. Suspicion of pancreatic lymphoma is a good example. However, in general, the pancreas can be a difficult place to obtain an adequate preoperative biopsy.

Because of the scirrhous nature of pancreatic tumors, biopsies and brushings are often negative. The decision for surgery is based on imaging and the behavior of the mass. Cancers tend to obstruct ducts and veins. It is important to inform patients and families that after an extensive and potentially damaging surgical procedure, a benign diagnosis is still possible. On the other side, a longstanding stent may predispose to a false-positive brush biopsy/cytology. The greatest importance of a biopsy now resides in establishing the diagnosis for palliative or neoadjuvant chemotherapy.

➢ Wisdom

A biopsy is not a prerequisite for pancreas resection.

Patients with pancreatic cancer are often stented prior to surgery in order to relieve jaundice. While the wisdom of this strategy is open to debate, you will still have to manage this situation as many patients arrive previously stented by our GI colleagues. Relieving jaundice does improve the patients' well-being and appetite. If you cannot operate immediately, this is a reasonable strategy. Stenting does, however, predispose patients to a potential unpleasant attack of acute pancreatitis, low-grade cholangitis and an increased postoperative infection rate. Careful surveillance of stented patients waiting for surgery is important to prevent any unplanned operative surprises. A major pancreatic resection in a patient with cholangitis can be a disaster. Check the INR and administer vitamin K; consider nutritional therapy in a debilitated patient (remember A.O. Whipple).

The other downside to preoperative stenting is that it occasionally causes, what we have characterized as 'stent' cholecystitis. Bacterial contamination of the biliary tree and partial duct obstruction predispose to cholecystitis.

This may manifest itself from mild inflammation around the gallbladder during the Whipple procedure to frank suppurative cholecystitis. Pus in the gallbladder predisposes to postoperative sepsis.

➤ Wisdom

Don't operate on a patient with cholangitis.

Deciding how aggressive to be in a patient with pancreatic cancer is an age-dependent process for both surgeon and patient. Young patients and young surgeons are the most aggressive combination. It is easy to justify prosecuting an operation on a 50- or 60-year-old and hard to justify on a 90-year-old. After all, the cure rate is low and morbidity is high. As always, it is the in-between patients where decisions are difficult. Shortening a life is regrettable. Large tumors in elderly patients are best left alone as size is related to oncologic outcome. Be wary of doing any type of pancreatic head resection on a patient with portal hypertension and varices through the porta hepatis. Dissection and control of bleeding can become impossible.

➤ Wisdom

A young surgeon and young patient are an aggressive combination.

An old surgeon and old patient; not so much.

A preoperative triphasic CT scan is your roadmap to pancreatic head resection. It allows you to internalize the patient's anatomic vagaries before operating. It can show an accessory artery or an occluded coeliac axis.

Remember, your job as a good HPB surgeon is to know the patient's anatomy before operating on them.

Diagnostic laparoscopy can be useful when you are looking for a reason to avoid the operation. Patients with cholangiocarcinomas have a high incidence of peritoneal spread. The presence of ascites on imaging should always raise this possibility and any significant amount of peritoneal fluid should be sampled for cytology preoperatively.

 Wisdom

The preoperative CT is your map; look at it.

Controlling blood loss in pancreatic surgery

The portal venous circulation has the inconvenient reality of possessing higher pressures than other venous systems. This means that small errors can result in an impressive volume of bleeding; control can be problematic. The tripartite area of the splenic, superior mesenteric and portal vein (deep location and multiple tributaries) means bleeding takes on a different dimension. Above and below control is not possible and clamps are challenging to apply. Preparing for the worst requires pre-emptive wide exposure. In this way a vessel that starts bleeding can be sutured before it gets out of control. An extended Kocher maneuver should be done early so that hand pinching can be used to control portal venous bleeding during a Whipple procedure. The front and back walls of the vein are compressed and then suction can clear the field for repair. On the left side this means early exposure of the entire length of the inferior pancreatic body and tail. Remember that clips tend to rub off; tie the tributaries off the portal circulation. Suture ligatures offer extra added security.

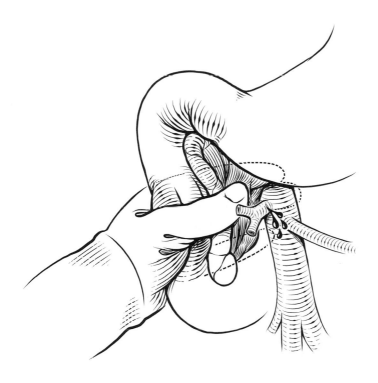

A major venous tear in an inaccessible location is always a significant concern. Early pressure control will allow for a short time-out and planning. This should include notifying the anesthesiologist and obtaining expert assistance. If it is coming from a cavity, a strategic small pack may allow temporary control. Dissecting around the area and even dividing the pancreatic neck can provide the wider exposure necessary for repair with fine Prolene® sutures. Circumferential control of all three veins or even rapid removal of a large tumor may be required to handle the situation.

Incisions

A midline incision suffices for most pancreatic operations. On occasion it has to be large. The pancreatic body may extend above the costal margin and the lower duodenum may extend to the pelvic brim. The deep position of the pancreas requires a longer incision to prevent key-hole exposure in large patients. Thick abdominal walls that lack pliability, and barrel chests (your typical truck driver), can also limit exposure. Subcostal and flap incisions have their place in selected circumstances. Skilled and experienced surgeons can utilize a good retractor system and small incision to effect; however, when trouble is anticipated or arrives, the incision must be rapidly expanded. Laparoscopic resection can offer a solution in selected patients.

Head of pancreas operations (Whipple)

The skilled performance of a Whipple procedure often defines what is a wise HPB surgeon. Just finding and evaluating the pancreas in a large patient can sometimes be a struggle. The omentum must be divided or reflected off the transverse colon and the right colon must be retracted inferiorly off the pancreatic head and right kidney. Keeping these structures clear of the area being exposed during any procedure can be arduous and is a task for your non-complaining retractor. A massive fatty omentum will torture you; remove it early.

An extended Kocher maneuver really gets things underway; this means getting all the way over to the aorta. The Kocher also starts at the common bile duct and ends under the SMV. The preliminary steps in a Whipple procedure need to be practiced and performed with care. The gonadal vein arising from the inferior vena cava is often close and damage can cause an annoying distraction. Comfort with the anatomy will eventually breed efficiency. It is useful to remember that as one dissects around the C-loop of the duodenum the superior mesenteric vein will come into view. This is a key landmark and can be followed to the neck of the pancreas. It is important to get on this vein and stay on it. Mesenteric traction can tear the gastrocolic trunk or middle colic vein resulting in some startling bleeding and staining of tissues that need to be dissected. These vein tributaries are often very delicate. It is reasonable to divide them early. The wide stump of the gastrocolic trunk should be suture ligated.

Real, above, below and side (splenic vein) vascular control of the portal venous system is usually not practiced unless a portal vein resection is planned or mobilization of the portal vein is required to address an uncinate tumour adjacent to the superior mesenteric artery.

 Wisdom

Only inattentive surgeons tear SMV tributaries.

A key early step is freeing the duodenum inferiorly under the mesenteric vessels. Three-dimensional anatomic confusion is the rule when dissecting the third and fourth part of the duodenum. It simply looks different from the left and right sides. The exact position of the uncinate process and portal vein are difficult to delineate from the left. Exposure here, without a major visceral rotation, is limited. Early connection of the duodenal and jejunal dissections will help orientation. Understanding how all these areas come together takes time with many 'explorations of the environment'. Watching will not develop the three-dimensional map that needs to be learned; mentor directed exploration will.

With practice the porta hepatis dissection will become familiar. We divide the common hepatic duct early and then clear over the top of the portal vein moving to the left. We also place a small Foley catheter in the divided hepatic duct to prevent any spillage of what is usually contaminated bile. A clamp may damage the end of the bile duct so is best avoided. The gastroduodenal artery (GDA) is of special significance. Dividing it opens the space above the pancreas. Clamp the GDA to evaluate the blood flow in the hepatic artery before dividing it. Obstruction of the coeliac axis may make the GDA the sole source of arterial blood flow to the liver. It must also be remembered that it is the change in the hepatic artery pulse/thrill that is essential to assess during on/off GDA clamping. Rarely, the common hepatic artery arises from the SMA and traverses the pancreatic head. Reconstruction of this artery may be necessary to proceed with resection.

➢ Wisdom

Beware the vasculopath; their hepatic artery may be GDA-dependent.

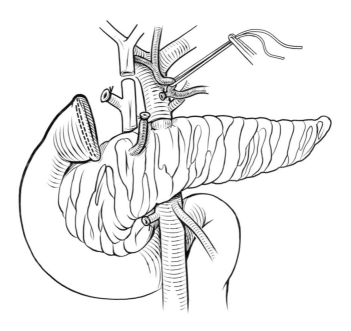

We generally like to divide the stomach before attacking the pancreatic neck. We divide it with a stapler and pack it out of the way under the left liver. When mobilizing the stomach be aware that it is now supplied exclusively by the left gastric artery. This artery needs your respect. Some HPB surgeons will divide the gastrointestinal tract after the pylorus (pylorus preservers), while others divide the distal stomach (classic). Reasons for selecting one option over the other include surgeon comfort and training, and the location of the tumour. While postoperative delayed gastric emptying is common with either approach, it is important to remember the utility of erythromycin as a prokinetic agent to treat this condition. Gastric emptying always improves with a little patience.

Dissecting the entire tunnel under the pancreatic neck should await completion of the porta hepatis dissection so that it can be attacked from both sides. Despite what is written, there are occasional vessels on the anterior surface of the portal vein. This dissection can be very easy or truly impossible. In a normal pancreas, the tunnel separates easily. If the tumor is close, it does not. Cancers tend to cause desmoplastic reactions in this area that fuse and pull surrounding tissue towards the tumor. Delineating this from tumor invasion can be difficult. Patience and persistence can usually result in a successful tunnel. Moving to the left side of the SMV/portal vein may provide a free pathway forward. This process cannot be forced.

Creating an 'invisible vein flap' can occur in the best of hands. This is a situation where when dissecting the tunnel from below, the right angle dissector skives a flap through the anterior wall of the SMV/portal vein. It initially bleeds a lot but when the angle dissector is removed, the flap closes and bleeding ceases. Repeated dissection in this plane just repeatedly opens and enlarges the flap. Eventually one may even recognize that the tip of the right angle dissector is in the lumen of the vein (you are looking at it through the vein wall — yikes!). The flap is not initially identified because it is behind the neck of the pancreas. To avoid creating the flap, keep the pressure of the right angle dissector tip upwards towards the posterior wall of the pancreas. If a flap is made, dissect in the other direction on a different line. On opening the pancreatic neck, the flap may be inapparent as it has sealed. Occasionally it has to be sutured.

➢ Wisdom

It's easy to skive the tip of your right angle dissector into the portal vein and create an 'invisible vein flap'.

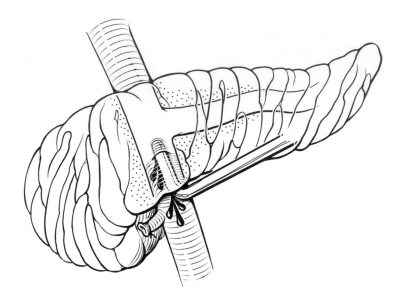

Dividing through the pancreatic neck can be a bloody affair, so we suture the four corners and use cautery over a Kelly. It is important to make this division 'square'. Oblique division in any plane will make the reconstruction more difficult. After neck division, an adhesed vein can usually be separated from surrounding tissues with gentle blunt dissection. If it has truly invaded the vein, a lateral vein wall resection may be required. Most of the time, placing a Satinsky clamp and removal of a small amount of the vein side wall is all that is needed. The vein may be narrowed 30-40% before a patch graft is necessary.

Removing the pancreatic head from posterior elements can be difficult in thick humans with large tumors. Energy devices can be very useful here but the pancreaticoduodenal vessels still need to be sutured. The uncinate process extends under the SMV; careful traction allows medial dissection to deliver it from under the vein. The posteriorly directed first jejunal vein branch is an excellent landmark for dissection above the uncinate. Attention must be paid to the position of the superior mesenteric artery. Feel for it, identify it and dissect it. The artery can bulge out from under the portal vein, quite far to the right, and is at risk of damage. We used to use a linear stapler on this area until a colleague stapled across the SMA. We don't do that anymore! Although this area is where HPB surgeons separate their talents, margins can still be positive despite best efforts.

➤ Wisdom

Look and feel for the SMA in the posterior dissection.

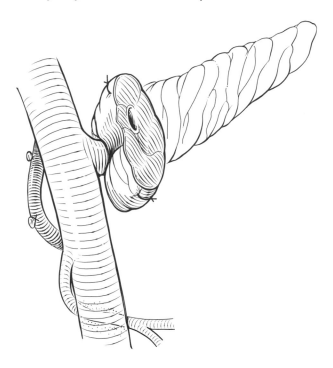

There are many reasonable pancreatic reconstruction methods. Dogma about which is the best seems unjustified. They can all leak. Trainees should be exposed to several techniques and master at least one. We feel that using interrupted rather than running sutures on any pancreatic connection is important. The loss of one suture then means a limited leak and not disruption of the entire suture line. Time must be spent on defatting the edges of the pancreatic stump so sutures are placed into real pancreatic tissue. In recent years we have had some success with pancreaticogastrostomies in patients with a soft normal pancreas. We then do not have to pretend that we can sew a 1mm pancreatic duct. With any of these pancreatic connections, we tend to place a whole row of individual sutures and then tie them at the end. This improves visibility for precise suture placement. The critical emphasis here is to be absolutely superb at one anastomosis, and possess others as back-ups in the rare situation that demands it.

➢ Wisdom

Running sutures change a leak into a disruption.

Don't sew fat!

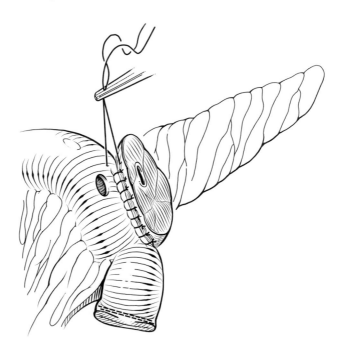

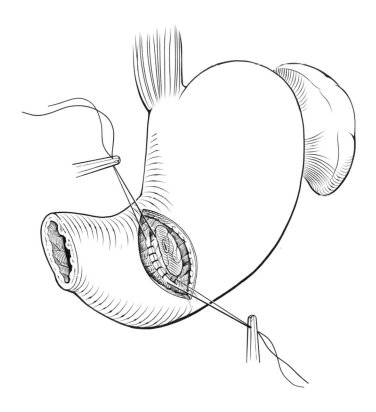

Learning how to place the reconstruction jejunal limb so that it lays easily without tension requires tricky three-dimensional thought processing. Kinking of the jejunal mesentery can cause lymphatic obstruction and bowel edema which can predispose to anastomotic leakage. The space through the right mesentery offers the most direct path. Remember to close the mesentery to prevent internal herniation of bowel. A CT scan of patients with pancreatic leaks often shows significant edema in this jejunal limb.

Gastrointestinal reconstruction also has significant surgeon variability. Most surgeons do not resect the antrum unless there is tumor encroachment. Duodenal dissection adds some work but sewing to duodenum is easier than stomach. It is a personal preference. If you do plan to preserve the duodenum, be sure to leave the vagal nerve supply intact.

The degree to which surgeons prosecute vascular resections varies from therapeutic nihilism to aggressive artery and vein resection and reconstruction. Whipple procedures do lend themselves to sleeve SMV/PV resections as 3-4cm of the vein is redundant after removing the pancreatic head. Notice that the portal vein is always kinked after the pancreatic head is removed. Each surgeon must work within their own comfort zone and always put the patient's interest ahead of any ego-driven behavior. Arterial resections are risky as any pancreatic fluid leakage can result in truly impressive arterial bleeding from erosion and disruption of the connection. Wise surgeons may consider doing a total pancreatectomy in this situation.

➢ Wisdom

Pancreatic juice is like acid to arterial connections.

Left pancreatic operations (distal pancreatectomy)

There are several points about the left pancreas that are important for HPB surgeons. The lack of intimate surrounding structures makes the left pancreas easier to operate. Early control of the splenic artery and vein offer a margin of safety. Most surgeries can be performed through a midline incision, but left subcostal incisions can be useful if a limited resection is planned. While it is always nice to preserve the spleen, this should not compromise the margins in a cancer operation. It is important to remember that the splenic vein on the left usually resides within a groove in the posterior pancreas so that the easiest dissection plane is around both. This is not the situation centrally, in the pancreatic neck, where the easiest dissection plane is found above the splenic vein (near the SMV/portal tunnel).

For most procedures, inferior mobilization of the splenic flexure of the colon is an important first step. This really clears the inferior border of the pancreas and exposes its relation to the spleen. The splenic artery, splenic vein, pancreas and fat at the splenic hilum can create a confusing meeting place. It is best to study the preoperative imaging to plan an approach to this area. It can be a no-go area if the tumor is adjacent to the spleen. You are also unlikely to preserve splenic vessels if they are interdigitated with the tail of the pancreas. Be humble and do a splenectomy when necessary. If there is any degree of splenic vein narrowing or obstruction, a splenectomy is mandatory.

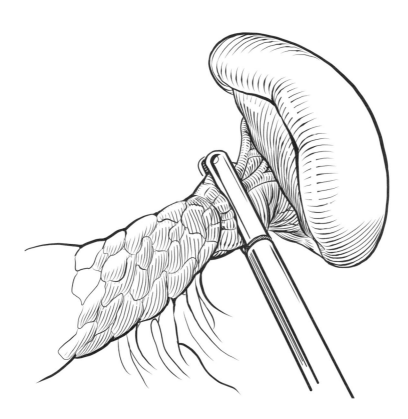

Leaving any remnant of pancreas in the splenic hilum is to be avoided as it may create a longlasting pancreatic fistula. Many body and tail tumors can be removed en bloc without central dissection. Stapling the pancreas with vessels attached is reasonable although purists would suggest that the pancreas and vessels should be taken separately. Saving the spleen is not a priority in an operation for invasive malignancy. However, for non-invasive tumors and cysts, preserving splenic vessels and the spleen is an elegant operation (laparoscopic or open).

The decision to preserve splenic vessels is often a personal choice. Taking the vessels and preserving the spleen on short gastric and left gastroepiploic vessels is well tolerated. Sometimes splenic infarcts may cause postoperative shoulder pain. These areas of spleen revascularize; we have not seen splenic abscesses. It is interesting that regional varices around the spleen are often observed on follow-up imaging. The patients develop gastroepiploic/left gastric arterial collaterals to the splenic short gastric inflow vessels. With the loss of the splenic vein the less compliant short gastric venous outflow cannot match the inflow so gastric varices develop. Gastric variceal bleeding has been reported. In a young patient, a vessel-preserving distal pancreatectomy is more of a consideration.

➢ Wisdom

Be humble and do a splenectomy when necessary.

When the cancer is close to the pancreatic neck and portal vein, a different approach is necessary. Approaching a tumor centrally and working retrograde after exposing the SMV/portal/splenic junction is reasonable. Dividing the neck of the pancreas can also provide comforting access to the splenic artery and vein. Early control facilitates the operation. The left adrenal gland may be involved with tumor and require en bloc resection. Rather than getting too distracted on an antegrade versus retrograde approach, perform a wide dissection and let the 'path of least resistance' guide your way.

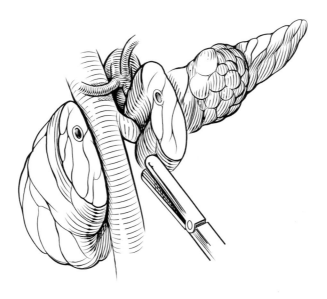

Endostaplers work great in open pancreatic surgery. Proximal and distal control of a splenic artery and vein is very effective. It is an instrument with the fidelity to get into a tight space. It is perhaps less necessary for pancreatic parenchyma. It is important when controlling the splenic artery that some navigation takes place. It is easy to mistakenly dissect the common hepatic artery. If in doubt, test clamp the perceived splenic artery prior to division, just as you would for the GDA during a pancreatic head resection. Widen your view, expose the porta and check your landmarks (lymph node 8a, left hepatic artery, gastroduodenal artery, etc.). Sewing the pancreatic duct has been shown to decrease leak rates. We also sew the stump with care, as if it is an anastomosis.

Laparoscopic distal pancreatectomy

Distal pancreatectomy is perhaps the most common HPB procedure to complete laparoscopically. Patient selection is important. Many of the indications are for premalignant lesions where local invasion is unlikely. Morbid obesity can make these procedures very challenging. Not having a large two-posted retractor requires some alternate strategies for retraction and exposure. First, we place large ports that allow the camera and staplers to be moved around to get the vision and angles right. We get the stomach out of the way early by suspending it from the anterior abdominal wall with tapes. This will also allow a little head-up, right-side down position to drop the transverse colon and splenic flexure. Energy devices create heat so care must be taken not to burn a spot on the colon that will leak down the road. Also, when taking pancreas off the splenic artery, beware of heating up the artery as it can create subsequent pseudoaneurysms.

 Wisdom

Beware of the heat produced by your energy device.

Wide exposure of the inferior border of the pancreas is the window to a successful operation. This should be done early with complete mobilization of the splenic flexure of the colon. Keeping the dissection near the spleen removes a remarkable amount of fatty omental tissue from this area and allows gravity to pull it out of the way. With great exposure, lifting the pancreas off Gerota's fascia and out of the retroperitoneum can be remarkably facile. The site of the tumor and location of vessels in the splenic hilum can help you decide to take the pancreas with vessels or not and whether a splenectomy is necessary. A slightly devascularized spleen on short gastric vessels causes no problems. It is, however, important to get the entire tail of the pancreas out and not leave a leaking remnant.

The splenic vein and artery can be dissected and encircled near the pancreatic neck as they are unlikely to be embedded in the pancreas at this location. The pancreas can then be stapled and the vessels dissected off for non-malignant surgical indications. Stapling the vessels separately in this proximal location is safest. For distal lesions with vessels embedded in the pancreas, it is probably best that they be stapled together.

Control of the pancreatic stump is an ongoing concern. We place the stapler carefully, close it slowly and leave it for a few minutes before firing. However, a thick pancreas may just not staple well. The stapler can crush the parenchyma leaving parts of the stump open for leakage. Finding and suturing the pancreatic duct or oversewing the entire stump is difficult (but not impossible) laparoscopically. Unless we have a soft flat pancreas that staples well, we feel that leaving a drain is worthy of strong consideration. Occasionally, the stapler will not close on a large rounded pancreas. The options here are to divide it laparoscopically with cautery or make a small incision and do it open through what we call the 'extraction site'.

 Wisdom

Drain a stapled pancreatic stump.

Central pancreas operations

A tumor that is in the pancreatic neck requires special consideration. It may not appear on imaging to invade vascular structures, but often does. Wide exposure of the central compartment is preferred. This allows assessment of resectability before too much dissection is performed. Resecting the portal vein is difficult with left or central pancreas resections as the vein is not redundant (as is the case after a pancreatic head resection). Resecting a pancreatic neck tumor may require dissecting into the head to obtain a negative margin. However, significant extension should best be treated with a Whipple procedure. Preserving pancreatic body and tail in a central resection requires consideration. A higher incidence of postoperative diabetes (10%) versus the risk of leakage from a soft pancreatic anastomosis remains the issue.

Completing a pancreatic operation

The completion of a pancreatic operation is a little different than other surgeries. Ensuring there is no ongoing bleeding should not be left to the end. It should be done carefully at each stage of the operation and then not revisited. Pawing around at the end looking for a bleeding source, or just checking anastomoses can cause problems. Delicate connections can be pulled apart. Leave them alone. Get your sponge count done early for the same reason. It is easy to misplace a sponge in these long multifaceted cases. Some surgical centres routinely do an on-table X-ray.

Drains should be placed very carefully for the same reason. Sometimes it is better to place the drains early when exposure is still good. Position your drain close to, but not right on, the stump or connection. Place it in a posterior dependent spot. There is no point in sucking right on a pancreatic connection (perhaps it will create a leak). It is also these deep areas where interventional radiologists have difficulty placing drains. Make the tract as straight as possible and laterally away from the wound. Be cautious not to lock the drain into the closing fascial suture. When doing your abdominal wall closure make sure these tubes are not displaced; a drain that slips into the pelvis offers little advantage.

Wisdoms

- *A biopsy is not a prerequisite for pancreas resection.*

- *Don't operate on a patient with cholangitis.*

- *A young surgeon and young patient are an aggressive combination. An old surgeon and old patient; not so much.*

- *The preoperative CT is your map; look at it.*

- *Only inattentive surgeons tear SMV tributaries.*

- *Beware the vasculopath; their hepatic artery may be GDA-dependent.*

- *It's easy to skive the tip of your right angle dissector into the portal vein creating an 'invisible vein flap'.*

- *Look and feel for the SMA in the posterior dissection.*

- *Running sutures change a leak into a disruption.*

- *Don't sew fat!*

- *Pancreatic juice is like acid to arterial connections.*

- *Be humble and do a splenectomy when necessary.*

- *Beware of the heat produced by your energy device.*

- *Drain a stapled pancreatic stump.*

Chapter 24

Pancreatic special circumstances

Turn your wounds into wisdom.
Oprah Winfrey

The leaking pancreas

A high index of suspicion for a postoperative leak is necessary for all patients with a pancreatic connection. A competent ampullary sphincter with higher pancreatic duct pressure can also cause distal pancreatectomy stumps to leak. Any postoperative concerns should be considered a leak until proven otherwise. Check the drain lipase on day 3 and only remove it if lipase levels and drainage volumes are low.

Perianastomotic drainage has proven benefit. Leakage control is important, but this is more likely from better surveillance. A drain that goes from clear to murky or shows high lipase/amylase levels should be taken as an early sign of leakage and the troops should be mobilized. Surgically placed drains often do not completely control a leak making percutaneously placed drains necessary. Smaller collections can be treated with antibiotics alone.

➢ Wisdom

A drain is the path to the soul of your pancreatic connection (if it looks ugly, it is).

Leakage can present as simply as delayed gastric emptying or as complicated as cardiorespiratory collapse. Early recognition and rapid treatment remains critical in the reduction of subsequent mortality. Our ability to salvage patients in the face of this problem has improved dramatically with interventional radiologists and critical care specialists becoming key players in any HPB program. The rule of Ts maps a universal strategy for a leaking pancreas: pay aTtention, Tube in the nose (nasogastric tube), Tube in the collection (percutaneous drain), TPN (hyperalimentation), Tazocin (broad-spectrum antibiotics) and Transfer to the ICU (if unstable).

 Wisdom

Remember the rule of Ts.

Unfortunately, leaking can turn into bleeding with blood vessel erosion and pseudoaneurysm formation. Any amount of blood in drains or the NG tube is a 'herald bleed' and should be investigated. Bleeding can be intraluminal, extraluminal or a combination of both. An early postoperative unstable patient that does not immediately improve with resuscitation should be returned to the operating room. In less dramatic circumstances, CT angiography followed by angiographic embolization is best. With any bleed from the common hepatic artery (GDA) stump, it is important to maintain blood flow to the liver. This artery should only be embolized in drastic circumstances or when accessory blood supply is present. An endoluminal stent will stop bleeding and maintain flow. It is essential that the hepatic artery remains open because your portal dissection has removed all collaterals. Complete hepatic artery occlusion, in this circumstance, can lead to full-on hepatic failure and patient mortality. If there is an intraluminal bleed, an attempt at gentle endoscopic control is reasonable.

Patients with widespread contamination should be returned to the operating room for washout. If there is disruption of the pancreatic anastomosis, a completion pancreatectomy may save the patient's life. At this stage, many patients are already in the ICU and requiring significant support. In these circumstances, inviting a colleague's opinion is always a good idea.

Borderline resectable

Pancreatic head tumors may be deemed 'borderline resectable'. The problem here is that there are many different definitions of 'borderline'. This can vary from the tumor touching the portal vein, to 180° involvement, to complete vein occlusion. Short segment involvement of the hepatic artery has also been delineated borderline. Most surgeons would agree that involvement of the superior mesenteric artery makes the tumor clearly 'unresectable'. The definition of borderline is very much dependent on how aggressive the surgeon feels. Of course, this completely misses the point, which is to try to determine whether a surgical intervention will be meaningful to the patient. With the advent of improved neoadjuvant systemic chemotherapy, tumors can shrink and/or borders can become sterile. Our own philosophy is that if the vein is significantly indented, neoadjuvant chemotherapy is wise. Many programs are now using neoadjuvant chemotherapy routinely for all patients and this may become the standard of care. Developing a friendship with your local medical oncologist will make this process work and prevent fisticuffs.

 Wisdom

Make a chemo buddy — your patients will thank you.

Ampullary resection

Circumstances may arise where a full Whipple procedure is not necessary. Very small or *in situ* tumors of the ampulla can be resected locally. This is especially indicated in the comorbid patient, although the potential for problems is still relatively high. The key investigative tool to assess the ampulla is endoscopic ultrasound. It can be particularly useful, in delineating the depth of invasion and how far the tumor extends into the bile duct.

To perform this operation successfully, it is important to mobilize the head of the pancreas and duodenum as much as possible with an extended Kocher maneuver; the right colon must be moved out of the way. The duodenum is held forward with posteriorly placed sponges, behind the pancreas. After opening the duodenum, one will note a very redundant appearance of the duodenal mucosa. The surgical appearance is different than endoscopic as there is no insufflation. Stay sutures can improve visibility by pulling duodenal mucosa out of the way. The ampulla can be found as a small nubbin by gentle finger palpation. The resection should include the bowel wall, ampullary complex, and a small amount of pancreas. The dissection needs to go deep. Reconstruction with a meticulous anastomosis of the pancreatic duct and common bile duct to the duodenal wall is essential. Dilated ducts make this process much easier. Think of making a watertight connection; simply tacking the edges together is not adequate. The duodenal wall is redundant so closure is usually straightforward.

Checking a margin is reasonable but doing a lot of margins will not make up for the fact that this is an inadequate operation for most invasive cancers.

➢ Wisdom

Reconstructing after an ampullary resection requires an ANASTOMOSIS.

Extensive margin checking will not save a bad operation.

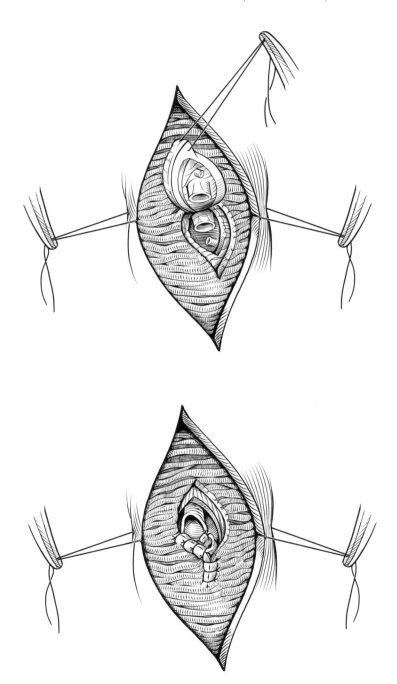

Enucleating pancreatic tumors

A local approach to removing some low-grade neuroendocrine tumors and premalignant cystic lesions is acceptable. While the morbidity and mortality are significantly less than in a resection, this should not change the indications for surgery. Enucleation can be more difficult than it appears. Localization of small tumors may require time spent with palpation and ultrasound, especially for lesions within the head of the gland. Digging into the pancreatic parenchyma always causes a certain amount of bleeding. Damage to the pancreatic duct guarantees a prolonged fistula and even without this a leak may still occur. Lesions in the tail should probably undergo a limited laparoscopic resection as morbidity here is low. Mandatory closed suction drainage will usually control any leakage and prevent sepsis. If the lesion is close to the pancreatic duct on preoperative imaging, enucleation is probably not the best approach.

Laparoscopic enucleations are a reasonable option for accessible benign pancreatic tumors. Good ultrasound skills are essential for accurate identification.

 Wisdom

Enucleations leak.

Pancreatic cancer palliation

In practice it may be impossible for pancreatic surgeons to 'do no harm'. HPB procedures have a remarkable capacity to hurt patients both in the short and long term. As cure rates for pancreatic cancer resection are dismally low, 'doing harm' should always be on a surgeon's mind. There is little worse than taking time from a patient or rendering them a hospital invalid for their remaining days.

Palliation remains the most common treatment of pancreatic cancer. The three main palliative problems for pancreatic head cancers are biliary obstruction, gastric outlet obstruction and pain. Historically, surgeons have addressed these problems to variable effect. Invasive operations on incurable patients are becoming increasingly suspect. Purely palliative surgeries, including bypasses, should only be applied to real or impending problems. Segment 3 bilioenteric anastomoses or Longmire procedures are largely of historical interest. Our endoscopic colleagues can usually do a reasonable job with stents at significantly less risk. Chemotherapy is proving increasingly effective in extending life; any procedure with or without complications may derail or delay this effective line of treatment.

➢ Wisdom

Don't delay chemotherapy by doing a 'heroic' operation.

An operative 'no go' from advanced local disease or unrecognized metastases represents a special circumstance. A delay in chemotherapy is already inherent in this situation. The patient usually has a biliary stent in place. We tend to move forward with a double bypass in younger robust patients with locally unresectable invasive disease, rather than metastatic disease. In other words, patients with a longer palliative time-line. If there were any problems with biliary stenting or if the tumor is already encroaching on the gastric outlet, we are more likely to perform a biliary/gastrointestinal bypass.

Sensory fibers from the pancreas transit the coeliac plexus. Chronic pancreatic pain can be effectively controlled with coeliac plexus blocks. At surgery, this can be done by injecting 10-20cc of 50% ethanol around the coeliac plexus. We use a two-person technique where the syringe is connected to the needle with flexible IV tubing. One person can then place the needle with good control and the other do the injection. This allows careful evaluation for blood vessel puncture by pulling back on the syringe.

Injecting any sclerosant into a blood vessel can have devastating consequences. At each site 3-5cc is injected before moving the needle. This can also be done effectively with upper GI endoscopic ultrasound.

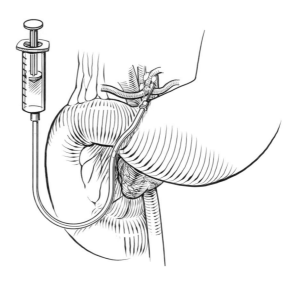

Stenting biliary obstruction can certainly improve well-being. However, it is an inexact science and many patients have repeated hospital admissions for pain and cholangitis. Endoscopically placed expandable metal stents have the best long-term patency. Hilar strictures are a special case where endoscopic stents often fail and percutaneous transhepatic drains are placed. They intermittently leak, block, and are work intensive; a general pain for patients. A surveillance program and low-dose antibiotics may improve the quality of life for these patients.

Transhepatic stents are more risky than their endoscopic counterparts. These stents have to be placed into Glissonian sheaths. While our interventional radiologists are very skilled at cannulating, even a non-dilated duct, anytime a Glissonian sheath is entered, blood vessel damage is possible. The inside of the sheath is 90% portal vein and perhaps more often than we realize the transhepatic stent traverses this vein. This may result in bleeding or clotting of the vein. Nothing too dramatic. However, if the catheter traverses the hepatic artery and into the duct, arterial bleeding and hemobilia can occur. This is heralded by significant pain and gastrointestinal hemorrhage. Thankfully, this is rare and can be readily corrected with angiographic embolization.

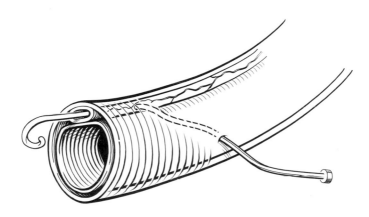

Autoimmune pancreatitis

Inflammatory conditions of the pancreas can mimic cancer. Autoimmune pancreatitis (AIP) often has a characteristic radiologic pattern with circumferential sausage thickening of the pancreas with little, if any, duct dilatation. However, a localized mass with biliary obstruction can also occur and appear exactly like a cancer. While an elevated IgG4 level can be useful in Type I AIP, it is far from diagnostic. It is critically important to look and ask patients for evidence of extrapancreatic inflammatory manifestations. This is not a part of Type II AIP disease which is confined to the pancreas. AIP patients can have a progressive course that is akin to an invasive cancer so following these patients, for a period of time, will not necessarily clarify the diagnosis.

In an ambiguous situation, a trial of high-dose steroids is a difficult decision. Prolonged stenting of a biliary stricture in a patient with an unclear diagnosis also has risk. If there is an underlying cancer, an opportunity at surgical resection can be missed. A truly multidisciplinary approach will result in the best possible diagnostic and treatment plan for these patients.

➢ Wisdom

Autoimmune pancreatitis is the great mimic.

Pancreatic cysts

If an HPB surgeon did not wish to operate frequently (a rare breed), he/she could spend their time immersed in the world of pancreatic cysts. A tidal wave of body imaging has resulted in a cascade of pancreatic cyst referrals. Most are small and of no consequence. Serous cystadenomas can often be recognized by their radiologic appearance and ignored. Even large microcystic tumors should be left alone. Mucinous cystadenomas are akin to biliary cystadenomas of the liver and should be removed because of their malignant potential. These cysts often have a thick wall and septations; they can be large and are more common in women. Side branch intraductal papillary mucinous neoplasms (IPMN) are generally smaller with thinner walls.

It may be impossible, on the basis of imaging, to know which of the three above diagnoses you are dealing with. Our radiologic colleagues will often label them side branch IPMNs; this does not make it true. The decision to operate is based on knowing the characteristics of the cyst and not necessarily the diagnosis. While there are probabilities involved here, it is only the pathologist who will give you the final diagnosis at the end of the day.

Generally, we remove cysts that are large (>3cm), have a thick wall or septations (probable mucinous cystadenoma) or have cancerous features (growth, mural nodules, pancreatic duct dilation). Also, if there is any suggestion of a main duct component (mixed IPMN), resection is indicated. Endoscopic puncture and cyst fluid analysis for CEA level and mucin can be useful in ambiguous cases. If one can prove a suspicious cyst is likely serous (low CEA level), surgery and surveillance are unnecessary. The presence of mucin, by itself, is not an indication for removal. This is especially true in elderly comorbid patients. Cyst fluid cytology is almost always negative and so rarely useful.

Most patients with pancreatic cysts are followed with serial MRI/MRCP scans so that repeated doses of radiation do not become an issue. How often and for how many years they should be followed is an unanswered question. Endless scans create expense and anxiety where risk is often small. At some point with small stable cysts, surveillance should stop; this point has yet to be defined. Size, growth rate, malignant features and age of the patient are all factors. A patient's comorbidity is a relative factor as some of these patients may risk an operation if there is a high likelihood of invasive cancer.

If you are going to follow someone, you have to have a trigger to operate. 'Death by imaging' is a real syndrome where we just continue to image and never intervene. There has to be a plan and the patient must be on board with this plan.

Some benign cysts can be effectively enucleated either open or laparoscopically. This is not an option if malignancy is considered possible.

➤ Wisdom

'Death by imaging' is real; have a trigger to operate.

ERCP complications

Your GI colleagues doing ERCPs may occasionally require your magnanimous help. Acute pancreatitis is a frequent complication, especially If they are playing with normal ducts or the sphincter of Oddi. It can be quite severe. Full-on necrosis of the pancreatic gland in a young patient with no real pathology is a tragedy.

A less common problem is perforation at the sphincterotomy site. The ampulla normally has a longish course through the duodenal wall so that the cut through the sphincter stays within the wall. If the cut is too long (like a sphincteroplasty) or the length of the ampulla in the wall is too short, a posterior perforation may occur. Most often this results in pain and some retroperitoneal air on CT. It is reasonable to admit the patient, cover with antibiotics and wait. Some of these will have a full-on duodenal leak. These patients will demonstrate retroperitoneal fluid on their imaging. If the collection localizes to the area around the duodenum, a percutaneous drain will work. Free perforation with sepsis may require a laparotomy washout and drainage. There is a well-described classification for post-ERCP perforations; however, clinical common sense based on repeat patient examination is the wise old standby.

Other perforations may occur including common duct or bowel. If a perforation occurs in a patient waiting for a Whipple procedure, proceeding directly to resection may be the best option if it is picked up early and the patient is not septic.

Sphincterotomy can result in bleeding. A repeat endoscopy can fix this problem. For the rare patient where bleeding does not stop, control at surgery should be done with a transduodenal sphincteroplasty.

Wisdoms

- *A drain is the path to the soul of your pancreatic connection (if it looks ugly, it is).*

- *Remember the rule of Ts.*

- *Make a chemo buddy — your patients will thank you.*

- *Reconstructing after an ampullary resection requires an ANASTOMOSIS.*

- *Extensive margin checking will not save a bad operation.*

- *Enucleations leak.*

- *Don't delay chemotherapy by doing a 'heroic' operation.*

- *Autoimmune pancreatitis is the great mimic.*

- *'Death by imaging' is real; have a trigger to operate.*

Chapter 25

Surgery for chronic pancreatitis

If fifty million people say a foolish thing,
it is still a foolish thing.
Anatole France

Seeking to cure a social disease (alcoholism) with surgery is a dubious undertaking. Wisdom may be designating your junior partner as the chronic pancreatitis expert. However, there are some patients with intractable pain from chronic pancreatitis that can benefit from a surgical approach. A desire to help should not force one's hand into an early operation. Complete alcohol abstinence, for an extended period of time, will help facilitate a compliant, motivated patient and improves results. Tobacco smoking remains the predominant driver for pain in these patients, and cessation is an absolute must prior to considering any operative intervention. A period of medical management with oral analgesia with the addition of local coeliac plexus blocks is also a good idea. After all, chronic pain often dissipates with a tincture of time and improved patient wellness from alcohol and smoking abstinence. Surgery is really an end-of-the-line therapy for chronic pancreatitis; often disappointing.

➤ Wisdom

Ongoing alcohol consumption and/or smoking is a good reason not to operate.

If someone does meet these criteria, then the next question is: resect part of the pancreas or internally drain the duct (resection vs. drainage vs. hybrid procedures)? Primary oncology surgeons likely favor a Whipple as that may be the only arrow in their quiver. A more nuanced approach is probably best. Disease that appears to be concentrated in the body and tail should be resected. A pancreas with a dilated duct can be drained into the jejunum. We routinely add a local resection of the pancreatic head (Frey procedure) to remove all impacted stones in this area and excise much of the increased neural hypertrophy driving the pain syndrome. Inflammatory masses in the head of the gland are seemingly rare, at least in North America. These procedures are often more fun for the surgeon than the patient.

Frey procedure

Full exposure of the pancreatic head, neck and body are the first step in this procedure. The initial challenge of a Frey procedure is to find the pancreatic duct. Refrain from attacking the pancreas with your cautery. Use your ultrasound machine and needle. When you get into the duct, leave the needle in place and use it as a guide to cauterize down into the duct. You can then open the duct up into the head.

➤ Wisdom

Use a needle to find the pancreatic duct and leave it in while opening the duct.

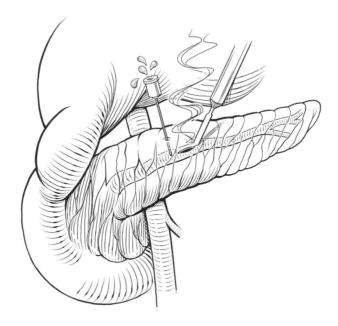

The gastroduodenal artery, on its course to the gastroepiploic artery, often becomes adhesed onto the anterior surface of the pancreas (just to the right of the neck). Don't forget to look for it and suture ligate either end or it will surprise you. It is often difficult to see in the inflammatory tissue on top of the pancreas.

> ## ➢ Wisdom

The gastroduodenal artery may be invisible as it crosses an inflamed pancreas.

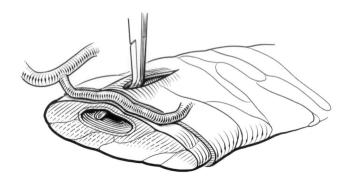

After the artery, the pancreatic duct takes an inferior turn deep into the head of the pancreas. It is at this point that a core of parenchyma must be removed. It can be a bit of a bloody affair but cautery will be your friend. There are often stones impacted duct deep in the pancreatic head. They are really calcium casts filling these dilated ducts and extending into side branches; they will resist removal and may have to be crushed. The common bile duct is close to this area. If you go medial you will get into it whether you wanted to or not. It is not a bad way to decompress an obstructed duct but be sure that is your intention before opening it.

➢ Wisdom

The common bile duct is close to the pancreatic duct in the head of the pancreas.

It is important that when you are coring out the pancreatic head that you leave a cuff of pancreas around the edges to sew. Don't get into the groove between the pancreas and duodenum as it will interfere with making a watertight connection. If you accidentally break through the posterior pancreatic capsule while coring out the head of the gland, you have two choices: 1) convert to a head resection/Whipple procedure; or 2) close the capsule with sutures, place a drain and accept a controlled fistula. We do our jejunal connection with interrupted sutures: it's good practice. We also put the heel of the bowel towards the pancreatic head (stapled end to the left), so if we have to come back to do a biliary bypass this piece of bowel can be easily pulled up to the bile duct. Just to show our confidence in this procedure, we often add an alcohol coeliac plexus block at the end.

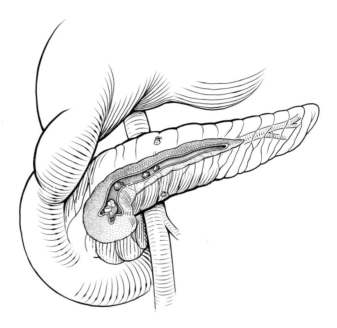

For patients with biliary obstruction, the duct may be decompressed within the parenchyma of the pancreatic head or with a separate hepaticojejunostomy higher in the porta hepatis.

Distal pancreatectomy for chronic pancreatitis

Resection is certainly an option for selected patients with chronic pancreatitis. Patients with disease that is confined to the left pancreas are ideal candidates. Indeed, patients with a history of mid-pancreatic trauma meet this criterion. If the disease process is extensive, this can end up being a left upper quadrantectomy including some stomach, adrenal and spleen. The real possibility of diabetes (if not already present) should be discussed with the patient preoperatively. Resection may also cure an annoying orphaned piece of distal pancreas following central pancreatic necrosis.

When approaching a patient with a chronically inflamed left upper quadrant pancreatic mass, take a very close look at the CT. Are there varices from splenic vein thrombosis (sinistral portal hypertension)? Does the inflammation involve the splenic flexure of the colon or stomach? Prepare yourself for difficulty. You can embolize the splenic artery preoperatively to reduce intraoperative variceal bleeding. Getting the spleen out of the left upper quadrant is key. It may be fused to the diaphragm and stomach. Rapid removal with a sliver of stomach may be necessary to control bleeding. Beware of damaging or resecting part of the diaphragm. If necessary, remove the spleen through a subcapsular plane (leave the splenic capsule on the diaphragm). Because of inflammation, landmarks may be obscured; experienced assistance is mandatory.

➢ Wisdom

Beware of diaphragm damage during removal of inflammatory pancreas/spleen.

Whipple procedure for chronic pancreatitis

A Whipple and total pancreatectomy are options for aggressive surgeons. Patients with intractable symptoms and an inflammatory mass in the head are candidates. These can be very difficult operations where it might be reasonable to employ two HPB surgeons. Often ruling out cancer in these patients is the rationale for a resection.

Chronic pancreatic pseudocysts

Pseudocysts in patients with chronic pancreatitis are not the same as those in the acute situation. They are often associated with fibrous stenosis of the main pancreatic duct. There is often no necrosis and they are less inclined to spontaneously resolve. They also tend to be smaller. Persistent symptoms may necessitate a surgical approach. Partial resection can be combined with a duct drainage procedure. It is important to discourage external drainage of chronic inflammatory pancreatic cysts, as an ongoing fistula may be the result.

 Wisdom

Chronic pancreatic disease does not like external drains.

Pancreatopleural fistulas

Rarely, chronic pancreatitis can produce a fistula tract into the pleural cavity with a resulting pleural effusion. The most likely presentation to the HPB service is persistent drainage of high lipase fluid through a chest tube. MR imaging may show this tract which extends through the diaphragmatic cura and into the chest. The first thing to do is nothing and wait for closure. However, persistent pressure may force intervention. Occasionally, a skilled interventional radiologist can drain the tract through the stomach, rerouting the flow. If there is an associated pseudocyst, drainage of the cyst into the stomach may do the same thing. Surgery involves resecting the pancreas source; easier said than done.

Wisdoms

- *Ongoing alcohol consumption and/or smoking is a good reason not to operate.*

- *Use a needle to find the pancreatic duct and leave it in while opening the duct.*

- *The gastroduodenal artery may be invisible as it crosses an inflamed pancreas.*

- *The common bile duct is close to the pancreatic duct in the head of the pancreas.*

- *Beware of diaphragm damage during removal of inflammatory pancreas/spleen.*

- *Chronic pancreatic disease does not like external drains.*

Chapter 26

Severe acute pancreatitis (riding the bull)

In the midst of chaos, there is also opportunity.
Sun Tzu

Wear protective gear and hold on tight. Although pancreatitis is 90% a medical disease, there still remains a 10% surgical horror. The management of severe acute pancreatitis is largely an escalating prosecution of supportive care and medical treatments right up to the point when it becomes surgical. Defining that point, when to pull the surgical trigger, is fraught with uncertainty. Intervening too early or too late is associated with poor outcomes. Severe disease may be associated with a poor outcome regardless of your perfect timing! Treating these patients may take many months and even up to a year in hospital; setting expectations with the patient and family is important.

The inflammatory process

The severely inflamed pancreas can destroy its own blood supply, causing necrosis and then leak caustic pancreatic fluid. This initiates a process of more auto-destruction with a cycle of more leaking and more destruction. The body deals with this by creating a retroperitoneal inflammatory rind to contain the damage. After several weeks the rind has formed a 'pseudocyst' containing inflammatory fluid and dead tissue, i.e., necrosum. The modern name for this situation is 'walled-off necrosis'. The necrotic part of the necrosum is made up of dead pancreas and dead retroperitoneal fat. It often extends around the retroperitoneum through paths of least resistance (paracolic gutters, down the path of the SMA/SMV, and around the spleen).

It can insinuate into the leaves of small and large bowel mesentery and travel as far south as the pelvis. It is important to remember that the walls of the pseudocyst are made up of the structures around the pancreas including stomach, jejunum, colon, spleen, mesentery and, of course, blood vessels.

➢ Wisdom

The walls of a pseudocyst are mostly bowel.

Significant acute pseudocysts do not usually form without some degree of pancreatic damage. Small pseudocysts resolve without intervention. Early peripancreatic fluid collections are common in pancreatitis and also do not require intervention. It is important to realize that even large non-infected necrosums can also resolve without intervention in sometimes minimally symptomatic patients. Decision making is not just a radiological review; you must actually look at the patient and monitor their pace of recovery or deterioration. It is important to recognize that the retroperitoneal process of transforming fluid collections to walled-off necrosis is dynamic and changes week to week.

Treatment decisions in necrotizing pancreatitis

The treatment of necrotizing pancreatitis has undergone a revolution in the last several decades. A very high mortality rate has decreased dramatically to less than 5% in high-volume centers. Timely intervention, at least 3 weeks after the onset of pancreatitis, and a single complete debridement are the new features of treatment. Most surgeons will acknowledge that improved critical care support is also a key factor.

➢ Wisdom

Intervening too early or too late is associated with a poor outcome.

The dictum of multiple repeat debridements with open packing has given way to a single clean-out of most necrotic material with drainage and abdomen closure. The idea of treating a walled-off pancreatic necrosum with percutaneous drainage alone has thankfully been abandoned. It does not drain this thick necrotic tissue and it infects any previously non-infected cavities.

The decision regarding when to operate is largely based on the trajectory of the patient's recovery. It is, therefore, important that the pancreatic surgeon be involved from the beginning. Early on, inflammation behaves like sepsis, up to and including hemodynamic instability, respiratory failure and renal insufficiency.

The 3-week wait rule does not apply to a patient in an early rapid downhill spiral, as bleeding and bowel ischemia/perforation can occur. The inflammatory process that is destroying small blood vessels in the pancreas can extend to regional bowel and other larger blood vessels. In other words, the severely decompensating patient within the 3-week window is most likely dying from an ischemic colon, biliary sepsis or abdominal compartment syndrome. Do not forget these diagnoses, because they will not forget you.

➤ Wisdom

Don't be dogmatic — you may still need early exploration in a deteriorating patient.

After this period, further demonstrations of sepsis, or hemodynamic instability, can initiate a surgical approach. Positive blood cultures and/or air in the necrosum are good signs of a superimposed infection. More difficult, is the recognition of a stalled recovery where improvements slowly dwindle away and eventually cease (i.e., 'persistent unwellness'). This should also trigger surgical debridement. We have never endorsed the repeated needling and culture of these necrosums. If you put a needle into these cavities enough times, they will all become infected. We base our decision on the changing status of the patient. It has also become clear that the idea of infected necrosis should not drive care or intervention. The patient's condition and ongoing behavior must prompt care decisions.

Wisdom

A stalled recovery may be a pancreatitis surgery trigger.

Prophylactic antibiotics have not been proven beneficial in severe acute pancreatitis. However, later in the course of the disease, antibiotics are often instituted as empiric treatment for presumed infected necrosis. Similarly, prophylactic ERCP for severe biliary pancreatitis is not indicated. However, in the situation of biliary obstruction and sepsis/cholangitis it can be lifesaving. Injecting or placing a drain in the pancreatic duct should be avoided to prevent contaminating the necrosum.

Operating in the 'maelstrom'

The standard of care remains exploration through a generous anterior midline incision with meticulous removal of all dead material and wide external drainage. Easy to say, but harder to do. The first barrier is finding the cavity. Pressure from a large cyst may obstruct portal/splenic venous return resulting in significant inflammatory varices that simply will not stop bleeding until the cavity is decompressed and evacuated. In this case the surgeon has to have the courage to forge ahead.

➢ Wisdom

When dealing with an inflammatory pancreatic hell, keep going.

The inflammatory bomb in the upper abdomen may make navigating a nightmare. A key strategy here involves identifying where the bowel and blood vessels reside in the inflammation. The two most common sites for access to the necrosum (not the bowel lumen) are through the gastrocolic omentum (under the greater curve of the stomach) and through the left transverse mesocolon. A seeker needle can guide exploration and prevent tearing into the bowel bluntly. On-table review of the CT will provide a roadmap to navigate safe entry into the necrosum. Similar to other cases, the surgeon should have their route into the walled-off necrosis planned before the operation starts.

➤ Wisdom

Seek the necrosum with a needle, not the bowel with your finger.

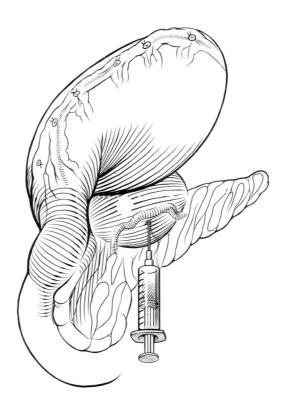

Once an opening is made, it can be gently expanded to allow for complete debridement of the cavity. Finger fracture and use of a sucker and ring forceps will allow a careful clean-out of the cavity. The right level of aggression when prosecuting the debridement is important. Too little and leaving residual dead tissue will slow recovery; too much and bleeding and bowel damage may occur. Pancreatic juice effectively destroys parenchyma but usually not blood vessels. When doing manual debridement these can often be felt as bands of tissue. Be gentle and leave them intact! While wide drainage through several large sump drains is necessary, we find the use of irrigation systems more suspect. They quickly create a direct irrigation stream between drain inflow and drain outflow. The body has the capacity to complete the debridement of residual necrosum. Significant bleeding should be dealt with by packing and your friendly neighborhood interventional radiologist (venous and arterial, respectively). Surgical control of bleeding from inside a necrosum is a tough game and it is better to leave a little dead tissue than debride the anterior wall of the portal vein.

After debridement, a pancreatic fistula is the rule. Fortunately, with a little patience, most will dry up spontaneously. This may take several months. During this stage any blood in the drain may herald a bleed from a pseudoaneurysm and require more help from your interventional radiologist. Indeed, this type of surgery should not be done without a radiologist at your side.

➢ Wisdom

An interventional radiologist is your bleeding pancreatic partner.

Transgastric debridement

New options for primary debridement are available. For well-developed necrosums confined to the retrogastric area, a transgastric approach through the posterior stomach wall has the advantage of creating an internal, rather than external, fistula. We perform an anterior gastrotomy and enter the cavity directly through the posterior stomach wall. This can be surprisingly difficult in an oddly placed walled-off necrosis. Use a seeker needle and suture the cyst wall to the stomach as early as possible as it can drop away. After debridement we complete circumferential sutures to prevent postoperative bleeding and leakage. Do not perform this approach for cavities that extend away from the stomach as it may be impossible to do a complete debridement. It is possible to do this transgastric debridement with a minimally invasive approach.

This same approach can now be completed endoscopically by motivated gastroenterologists. It is only successful with repeat sessions of endoscopic debridement (average of seven sessions). An endoscopic approach loses the opportunity to get a reasonable biopsy of the cyst wall and rule out a rare cystic pancreatic tumor as well.

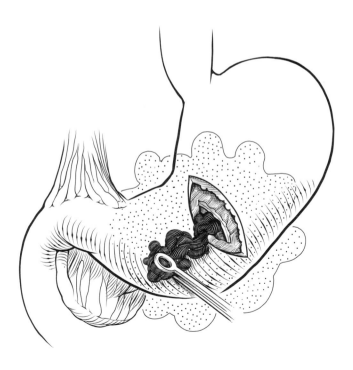

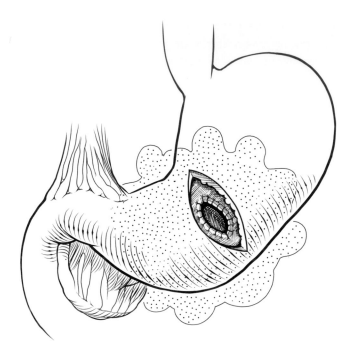

Other options for treatment

Despite a policy of single complete debridement, patients may have delayed recovery from isolated undrained/debrided areas. In this circumstance a local approach may prove satisfactory. This is particularly true in the flank where a paracolic collection can be cleaned out and drained locally. Positioning the patient on their side with the table broken will open this space. The colon is at risk of damage with a flank approach. This is perhaps the situation where a preoperatively placed percutaneous drain is useful. It offers a trail to the cavity that does not go through the colon.

➤ Wisdom

The flank is a window to a paracolic collection; break the table and open the window.

A primary flank approach to debridement is well described with VARD (video endoscopic retroperitoneal debridement). With long instruments and a long scope, it is possible to get a good central debridement from the flank. However, if the necrosum extends to the opposite side or elsewhere, it can be unreachable. Using laparoscopic tools and a scope to explore this space is the mantra. A frozen abdomen from previous surgery may make this approach the default (i.e., after a decompressive laparotomy for abdominal compartment syndrome).

➤ Wisdom

A drain can show you the money (follow the trail).

Pancreatic fistulas that do not close may require surgical intervention, but certainly not before 2-3 months. The fistula tract is internalized into a Roux limb of jejunum. Make the tract as short as possible when creating your connection; long connections lead to high pathway pressures and subsequent stenosis and re-accumulation of the pseudocyst.

Patients with central pancreatic necrosis may be left with an orphan disconnected left pancreas: a vascularized and isolated piece of pancreas towards the tail ('El Diablo'). This can cause pain, recurrent pancreatitis and pseudocyst formation. A difficult resection here, often including the spleen, can resolve these symptoms and bring the patient back to health.

The 'step-up approach' to treating pancreatic necrosis has level I supportive evidence so deserves mention. This technique involves placement of drains and minimally invasive techniques for debridement: endoscopic posterior gastric and videoscopic flank debridements. The results show a significant reduction in new-onset organ failure, fewer incisional hernias and less diabetes. It highlights one critical point. When you take these patients to the operating room for an open debridement you often make them significantly worse before they get better. Minimally invasive approaches cause much less surgically related trauma. If you are at an institution that has dedicated endoscopists and radiologists that are willing to do multiple procedures and take some responsibility for patient care, you should definitely consider this option. Sadly, these services are often rotational with the motivated parties often not 'on-service'. While some patients with minimal necrosis may get better with percutaneous drainage alone, most require step-up debridement, including surgery.

➢ Wisdom

Open pancreatic debridement can make patients worse before they get better.

A patient may present with a longstanding symptomatic pseudocyst with little or no necrotic debris. They have pain and an inability to eat from functional and mechanical gastric outlet obstruction. These are the classical patients that general surgeons would wait 6 weeks and then operate. They are actually not that common; most lesions that are referred to as 'pseudocysts' by radiologists and physicians are actually walled-off pancreatic necrosum collections. A pseudocyst that is enlarging or narrowing/obstructing surrounding veins is a good reason to intervene. If the pseudocyst is adjacent to stomach or duodenum, it is probably best for the GI endoscopist to have a go at it. Sometimes transpapillary drainage is possible. If they fail or there is no window, a surgical approach is reasonable. Use the closest piece of bowel or use a Roux limb of jejunum. We sew all these connections.

Severe acute pancreatitis is a multidisciplinary type of disease. A functional team of radiologists, gastroenterologists, intensivists, and surgeons will get the best results. This must include a team leader that is willing to commit to care of these patients for months and months. This person is usually a surgeon.

Wisdoms

- *The walls of a pseudocyst are mostly bowel.*

- *Intervening too early or too late is associated with a poor outcome.*

- *Don't be dogmatic — you may still need early exploration in a deteriorating patient.*

- *A stalled recovery may be a pancreatitis surgery trigger.*

- *When dealing with an inflammatory pancreatic hell, keep going.*

- *Seek the necrosum with a needle, not the bowel with your finger.*

- *An interventional radiologist is your bleeding pancreatic partner.*

- *The flank is a window to a paracolic collection; break the table and open the window.*

- *A drain can show you the money (follow the trail).*

- *Open pancreatic debridement can make patients worse before they get better.*

Section VI

HPB extras

HPB surgery is not a silo of disease and operations. The very anatomy and pathology that we strive to understand necessarily pushes into all parts of the abdomen. It is impossible to do these operations without a comprehensive understanding of the entire intra-abdominal cavity. Similarly, the care of these patients extends into all corners of the hospital. It consumes a huge volume of resources. How the HPB team interacts with these different areas, including the administration, can define success.

Chapter 27

Other organs of the upper abdomen

Science is organized knowledge. Wisdom is organized life.
Immanuel Kant

One cannot be an HPB surgeon without a knowledge of the surrounding organs. They are hazards that must be understood, retracted or resected. Comfort with operating in these areas makes it possible to extend HPB surgeries to en bloc resections when necessary to obtain negative margins.

Duodenum

Hepatopancreatobiliary and duodenal surgery (HPBD) is perhaps a useful abbreviation. The duodenum is a natural part of an HPB surgeon's universe. It is intimate with the stomach, pancreas, ampulla and mesenteric vessels. The duodenum is not just another piece of small bowel. It is a complicated three-dimensional structure that traverses around the mesenteric vessels. It is also largely retroperitoneal and difficult to expose. Only the anatomic HPB knowledge of all these surrounding structures allows safe surgery.

 Wisdom

The duodenum is NOT just another piece of small bowel.

The duodenum is the ever-disappearing organ. It begins anteriorly and visible. It ends posteriorly and invisible behind a great mass of mesentery and bowel. It effectively becomes part of the retroperitoneum. Any operation on the duodenum requires reflecting the right colon and its mesentery away and extending a Kocher maneuver to bring the duodenum up where it can be seen.

➢ Wisdom

Deliver the duodenum from the retroperitoneum.

A duodenal incision should only be as large as it needs to be. The duodenum flattens if it is opened too far, making reconstruction a challenge. When looking for something (bleeding ulcer), it's better to create two small incisions than splay the duodenum wide open.

➢ Wisdom

Large duodenal incisions end up looking like 'moss on a rock'.

The actual duodenal wall is robust with a good blood supply, but no mesentery. It is also a fairly wide segment of bowel that does not stricture easily; a duodenotomy can often be closed vertically. A duodenotomy tube is for your father's generation — if you sew it properly, the duodenum will not 'blow out' or leak. Once the duodenum is opened it is essential to orient to the ampulla of Vater. It can be surprisingly hard to find the ampulla and requires a lot of palpation and probing. Its position is variable and it can occasionally be found quite distal in the third part. You can also squeeze the gallbladder and look for bile (or open the cystic duct and pass a small catheter distally into the duodenum). The minor duct of Santorini can be a beast to find. Your friendly endoscopist can always help you with a preoperative stent.

 Wisdom

Think 'beware the ampulla' as you navigate the duodenum.

Surgeons may come to treat every duodenal tumor with a Whipple procedure and this is a shame. Tumors that are on the lateral duodenal wall can often be removed without pancreas. Gastrointestinal stromal tumors (GISTs) are a good example of a duodenal tumor that does well with local resection. Below the ampulla it is relatively simple to remove the entire third or fourth part of the duodenum without transgressing the pancreas. Above the ampulla the duodenal connection with the pancreas is much tighter and while removal is possible it is much more difficult (pancreatic head-preserving duodenectomy).

After a distal duodenal resection (third and fourth part), staple off the duodenal end and then do the anastomosis as far away from the pancreas as possible (lateral side to side). Trying to sew the end of the duodenum in the groove next to the pancreas is difficult and prone to leak.

 Wisdom

Side-to-side connections fit the duodenum.

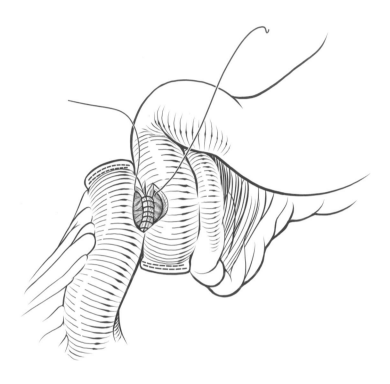

If there is significant bowel wall removed, the duodenum can be closed transversely. Duodenotomies that extend very medial into the pancreaticoduodenal vessels and pancreas are a concern. It can be difficult to get a watertight closure; bleeding and pancreatic damage are cause for heightened awareness. Pay attention to this during the resection stage; it is better to do a Whipple procedure than a medial duodenal wall resection close to the ampulla. Damage to the ampullary complex or a leak from pancreatic damage can create a nightmare scenario.

➢ Wisdom

If you get into the pancreas, think Whipple.

Operating on the fourth part of the duodenum is awkward as it is in a tight area. Success requires good exposure and good exposure requires complete rotation of the colon and small bowel mesentery superiorly. The trauma surgeons have a name for this which HPB surgeons do not need to know. Resection of the distal duodenum and part of the uncinate process may be possible without resorting to a Whipple. The mesenteric vessels are close and local invasion is common.

Duodenal diverticula are common but rarely cause problems. They sit in or around the ampullary complex; any type of surgical approach is hazardous. They are often confused with duodenal perforations in the patient who gets emergency CT imaging for non-specific abdominal pain. Duodenal diverticula have normal walls, no associated inflammation, free air or free/retroperitoneal fluid. Stay away.

➢ Wisdom

A duodenal diverticulum is not your problem.

Colon

The colon can be a sad part of many HPB surgical operations. It can be involved in gallbladder and pancreatic inflammation or cancer. Its blood supply can be compromised during an HPB operation.

The right colon is very much in the way of pancreatic surgeons and the hepatic flexure must be mobilized inferiorly to gain consistent exposure. A localized right colon cancer can involve the duodenum. Much of the duodenal wall can be resected in an en bloc resection before a Whipple resection is required. Pancreatic cancer Involvement of the colon is not a contraindication for en bloc resection. Indeed, removing the right colon makes things easy.

The transverse colon can be intimate with an inflamed pancreas. Damage during debridement is easy; the colon is always close. Extensive pancreatic inflammation may thrombose vessels in the mesocolon, effectively killing the adjacent colon. An unpleasant colon resection may save a life. If the perforated colon cannot be removed from the inflammatory mass, a loop ileostomy with colon lavage and drainage is a bail-out procedure.

The left colon/splenic flexure has to be moved to see the pancreatic tail, otherwise you are in a deep, dark bleeding hole. A pancreatic tail cancer can include colon. Again, en bloc resection should proceed without a second thought.

It can be a nice social event having your colorectal colleague in for a visit but the reality is that any colon that crosses your territory is fair game.

➢ Wisdom

The colon is fair game for an HPB surgeon hunting.

Stomach

With the demise of ulcer surgery, the stomach is a much less operated upon organ. It is quite thick and robust (it takes a stitch well). The mucosa is redundant and loosely attached to the submucosa. It has a four-artery blood supply so is difficult (but not impossible) to devascularize. Its blood supply is shared with the omentum (gastroepiploic), spleen (short gastric vessels), liver (left gastric) and pancreas (right gastric). You can remove large parts of it with minimal physiologic derangement.

Wisdom

The stomach can take a stitch.

With a Whipple procedure, two of three vessels are divided so retaining the remaining left gastric vessel is critical. Similarly, if leaving the spleen on short gastric vessels only (Warshaw procedure), it is important to preserve the left gastroepiploic artery. This artery has been shown in both CTA and MR studies to deliver the majority of the blood to the spleen when the main splenic artery is occluded. We do not divide the omentum under the stomach as this will lead to significant devascularization. Instead, we prefer to enter the lesser sac by reflecting the entire omentum off the transverse colon through this avascular plane.

The antrum with its G cells was traditionally thought to be ulcerogenic. Hence, the original Whipple procedure always included an antrectomy. We routinely leave the antrum and place the patient on a proton pump inhibitor (PPI) indefinitely. We have seen marginal ulcers in patients who omit this treatment.

Sewing jejunum to stomach is not tricky but it is important to note that the stomach does not stretch as much as small bowel so the opening should be made slightly larger than the jejunum. It also has a thicker wall that can entice learners to take bites that are too large. Antecolic versus retrocolic connections seem to make little functional difference in most patients.

Spleen

The spleen is one of those rare dual blood supply organs that can be a pleasure to operate on. While the main splenic artery and vein are dominant, it is amazing that the small short gastric vessels and left gastroepiploic artery can take over in a pinch. The spleen is tucked into a difficult corner of the left upper quadrant and is partly retroperitoneal behind a covering of stomach and colon. The operating key here is to release it from these surrounding organs and bring it to the midline.

Not many spleens are removed these days. Our trauma colleagues embolize most damaged spleens and hematologic indications for splenectomy are less common. This leaves HPB surgeons as the last practitioners of any significant volume of splenectomies. This is reasonable, as to know the tail of the pancreas is to know the spleen.

Removal of a normal spleen is a regular part of any distal pancreatectomy for cancer and exposure is the same. There are several tricks that will make life easier. Separate the spleen from the stomach early by taking down the short gastric vessels. Energy devices are great for this. Be sure to get right around the top of the spleen and start the peritoneal dissection behind. Textbooks talk about dividing the splenorenal ligaments, but perhaps they mean the peritoneal sweep under the spleen. Dividing this peritoneum is the key to splenectomy. It is usually unseeable, even with medial retraction of the spleen. Work from above and below, feel it with your fingers, and angle the cautery tip. Often though, you have to take a long pair of scissors and cut the peritoneum blindly! This opens the plane above the kidney/adrenal and allows the spleen and tail of the pancreas to come forward. This is one of the few times when an HPB surgeon can comfortably get their hand around the organ they are operating on.

➢ Wisdom

Divide the 'unseeable' peritoneum to release the spleen.

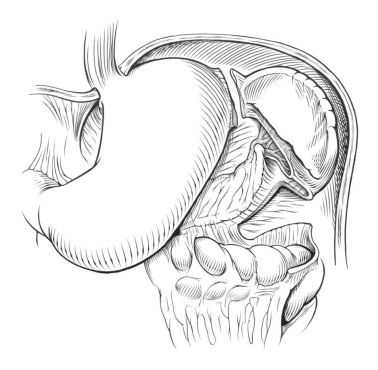

If it is just the spleen you want, look at the preoperative imaging to place the tail of the pancreas in relation to the splenic hilum. If it's away, proceed with the stapler. If the pancreatic tail nuzzles into the spleen you need to dissect the hilum to protect its integrity. Many times, surgeons just staple across the pancreatic tail (without knowing it) and this adds the risk of a pancreatic leak. If at any time, in a splenectomy, you start to get excessive bleeding, pull it up and staple the hilum; it happens!

> ➢ **Wisdom**

The pancreatic tail is a critical structure in splenectomy.

When taking out an enlarged spleen or one with splenic vein thrombosis, always control the splenic artery first. Look for it on the superior edge of the pancreas. You can also occlude it preoperatively with angioembolization. In truly massive spleens, the entire hilar and short gastric vessels should be divided before splenic mobilization. Going at the hilum first is also a reasonable option when the spleen is unmovable from retroperitoneal inflammation and adhesions.

➢ Wisdom

Take the splenic artery first to decompress your splenic worries.

A laparoscopic approach offers distinct advantages for most splenectomies in terms of visualization and patient comfort.

Splenectomy for splenic vein thrombosis and sinistral portal hypertension can be brutal surgery. These patients often have longstanding inflammation from chronic pancreatitis or an episode of severe acute pancreatitis. Extensive retroperitoneal inflammation in combination with high venous pressures and varices means trouble. Bleeding from gastric varices can often be controlled endoscopically with glue. Surgery is a last resort; consider splenic artery embolization instead and if you do plan to operate, embolize the spleen preoperatively.

Kidneys and adrenals

Knowing the base of your operative box Is important. The kidneys and adrenals sit at the bottom unseen and unloved. They can rough you up, every once in a while, if you do not show them some respect. You may also be asked by a colleague to move aside your beloved organs (liver and pancreas) to expose these deep monsters.

The right adrenal can stick to the back of the liver and cause a surprising amount of bleeding. Leave it in the retroperitoneum. A large tumor of the adrenal can often only be safely removed with right liver mobilization. Caval control and resection may be necessary. In a deep man this may require all your exposure tricks. The right kidney can occasionally be involved with pancreatic head tumors. It perhaps requires a bit more thought to remove it en bloc.

On the left side, the adrenal can easily be involved with a pancreatic tumor. Resection of the adrenal should not be given any pause if a negative margin can be obtained. This also could include the left kidney. Large tumors in the left upper quadrant are orphans waiting for your adoption if you are comfortable with the kidney and the concept of left upper quadrantectomy.

➤ Wisdom

The adrenals are an 'annoying piece of fat'.

Wisdoms

- *The duodenum is NOT just another piece of small bowel.*

- *Deliver the duodenum from the retroperitoneum.*

- *Large duodenal incisions end up looking like 'moss on a rock'.*

- *Think 'beware the ampulla' as you navigate the duodenum.*

- *Side-to-side connections fit the duodenum.*

- *If you get into the pancreas, think Whipple.*

- *A duodenal diverticulum is not your problem.*

- *The colon is fair game for an HPB surgeon hunting.*

- *The stomach can take a stitch.*

- *Divide the 'unseeable' peritoneum to release the spleen.*

- *The pancreatic tail is a critical structure in splenectomy.*

- *Take the splenic artery first to decompress your splenic worries.*

- *The adrenals are an 'annoying piece of fat'.*

Chapter 28

Dilated ducts and other oddities

Any fool can know. The point is to understand.
Albert Einstein

The high volume of intra-abdominal imaging being performed these days produces a lot of incidental findings in largely asymptomatic patients. Perhaps some of the most interesting of these findings are dilated ducts in the liver or pancreas. This, of course, raises the ugly spectre of cancer.

 Wisdom

A dilated duct requires an explanation.

A dilated duct in the liver could be a congenital nothing, but a small cholangiocarcinoma is definitely a consideration. MR imaging with delayed phases and contrast ultrasound should be completed to identify any mass. Patients with segment atrophy and 'duct crowding' often have a small low-grade cholangiocarcinoma that can be cured with resection. More proximal obstruction may result in atrophy of an entire lobe or sector with compensatory hypertrophy of the opposite side of the liver. It is usually more localized than primary sclerosing cholangitis (PSC). These patients also have no cholangitis symptoms, and no associated inflammatory conditions which distinguish them from PSC patients. If the obstruction looks relatively proximal, 'spy glass' cholangioscopy and biopsy can be enlightening. It should be recognized that duct dilation and atrophy takes time so if you are dealing with a cancer, it is likely to be low grade.

A dilated extrahepatic biliary tree with no mechanical obstruction is common, especially after cholecystectomy. Normal tumor markers, normal liver function tests and no mass on imaging should initiate a short course of surveillance only. If there is a suggestion of an obstructive cause, the patient should have an endoscopic ultrasound.

Congenital non-development of a sector or lobe of the liver is more common than readily appreciated. The imaging just looks 'unusual' and it takes some mental effort and landmarking of hepatic veins to recognize the small size of a specific area and compensatory hypertrophy of the other. Recognizing this preoperatively will prevent real anatomic intraoperative spatial confusion.

A dilated pancreatic duct, with or without atrophy, raises a number of possibilities. If the entire duct is dilated, think chronic pancreatitis or main duct IPMN. ERCP and endoscopic ultrasound should be performed to search for a patulous ampulla extruding mucin that is pathopneumonic of main duct IPMN. Keep in mind that all patients with main duct IPMN have some degree of chronic parenchymal inflammation within their pancreas and may also have had episodes of acute pancreatitis in the past. To make things even more uncertain, patients with imaging findings of chronic pancreatitis may have no history of pancreatitis or pain. Mucin in the duct is the key.

Main duct IPMN does not behave like side-branch IPMN; they have a very high rate of malignant degeneration and should prompt resection in all but the most elderly patients. Decades ago, surgeons had a complete misunderstanding of this entity and called it 'mucinous duct ectasia'. It was often treated as chronic pancreatitis to devastating effect!

Segmentally dilated pancreatic ducts raise the possibility of mixed IPMN, cancer or a remote injury from trauma. Be very suspicious, even if imaging does not show a mass. These are the types of patients where resection can cure.

You may see a number of patients with an annular pancreas in your office. If they obstruct, bypass them. Otherwise, leave them alone.

Pancreatic divisum is another oddity that gastroenterologists remain fixated upon. Pancreatic divisum and pancreatitis are both relatively common. We have yet to see any convincing evidence that they are in any way connected; leave pancreatic divisum alone. Sphincteroplasties of the minor ampulla of Santorini are a wonderful technical challenge but there is little real evidence they help patients.

➢ Wisdom

Developmental oddities of the pancreas are not your problem.

Sphincter of Oddi dysfunction/hypertension is an interesting diagnosis. There is likely no other entity that is more debated by gastroenterologists around the world. A formal diagnosis of hypertension in these often young, otherwise healthy females can only be achieved by formal endoscopic sphincter manometry. Thankfully these procedures are now rare in North America, as they are often (45%) accompanied by significant post-procedural pancreatitis. Given that the definitive treatment remains cutting the sphincter, perhaps proceeding to an ERCP-based sphincterotomy is a more straightforward option.

Wisdoms

- *A dilated duct requires an explanation.*

- *Developmental oddities of the pancreas are not your problem.*

Chapter 29

General surgery operations on cirrhotics

You know nothing, Jon Snow.
Game of Thrones

This is another job for your junior partner. Advanced cirrhosis is a good reason to do nothing (won't tolerate a haircut) and you can do most anything in a well-compensated cirrhotic. It is the in-between patient where wisdom in decision making bears its mark. Our hepatology colleagues can help us assess the liver function. The surgeon's job is to evaluate other comorbidities and search for portal hypertension and ascites. If they have either varices or significant ascites, elective operations are best avoided.

 Wisdom

Avoid elective surgery in patients with varices and ascites.

Gallbladders with varices growing up around their base are distinctly unpleasant. If you find yourself operating in this situation, remember you can always do less than a total cholecystectomy with removal of the stones. Vascular figure-of-eight sutures on the gallbladder stump are an excellent way to close off bleeding and get home. If you know about these varices ahead of time, consider a percutaneous drain and stone removal.

Wisdom

Varices on the gallbladder wall mean subtotal cholecystectomy.

Colon resections in patients with varices are also an 'un-fun' prospect. Energy devices (LigaSure™) can take some of the sting out of these problems, but large varices still need to be suture ligated (or at least secondarily clipped). Do not drop an anastomosis into an abdomen full of ascites and be aware that stomas created in cirrhotics leak ascites and often develop stomal varices. This is a no-win situation. It is perhaps best to let the colorectal surgeons deal with some of these cirrhotic issues including hemorrhoids!

 Wisdom

Colon surgery in an advanced cirrhotic is a no-win situation.

Hernias in patients with varices and especially uncontrolled ascites should be left alone. Medical control of ascites may allow a window for repair. A small amount of peritoneal fluid is not as big a risk as we once thought. However, resist the temptation to fix umbilical hernias in patients with advanced cirrhosis and ascites. If they rupture, it's an emergency and you can proceed 'blamelessly' in a situation where risks are high.

If you are forced to do an operation on a patient with significant ascites, it is reasonable to place a drain for temporary control. This allows the wound to peritonealise and avoid an ascites leak. Any uncontrolled fluid leak will eventually result in peritonitis. The drain can be removed in 3-4 days and the skin exit site sutured. Of course, maintaining fluid and electrolyte balance during this time can be a challenge.

Wisdoms

- *Avoid elective surgery in patients with varices and ascites.*

- *Varices on the gallbladder wall mean subtotal cholecystectomy.*

- *Colon surgery in an advanced cirrhotic is a no-win situation.*

Chapter 30

The HPB surgeon in trauma

*Trauma surgery is an art that combines decision-making
with technical and leadership skills.*
Asher Hirshberg

One reason you became an HPB surgeon was so you do not have to get up at night for trauma cases. So why are they calling you now? Trauma surgeons come in all shapes and sizes, and with varying experience; some may have very little liver and pancreas experience. They are pretty good with most bleeding, so if they are calling, it is likely to be bad. Remember that you are also good with bleeding and probably better when it is coming from the liver or pancreas.

The torn or shredded liver can be a dramatic event and your arrival will likely be in the middle of chaos. Simple solutions will have already been tried! Go back to your principles of exposure, inflow control and outflow control (EIO). Compressing the liver together with both hands may offer temporary control. Otherwise, pack, lengthen the incision and then get your fixed retractor in place. Do not bother to ask for a Rumel tourniquet as it will waste a lot of time with blank stares; just clamp the porta with a vascular clamp for your Pringle. Remember that continuous inflow occlusion in a trauma situation is not nearly as well tolerated as the elective liver resection patient. Forty minutes is perhaps the upper limit here. The CVP is already likely to be low, so don't ask the anesthetist to lower it. Outflow control in liver trauma means packing which can control hepatic venous bleeding.

Packing is less effective for arterial bleeding and is only a temporising move that allows you to get the patient to the angiography suite. Angioembolization is better than tying off a hepatic artery but should be used if the patient is too unstable to move.

Extensive disruption of the hepatic veins or vena cava may need a more dramatic solution. First, don't open a deep caval or hepatic vein injury that is contained. If bleeding forces your hand, total vascular exclusion may be necessary to obtain control above and below the damaged area. In this situation, clamping of the aorta must be utilized to prevent cardiac arrest in a severely hypovolemic and physiologically tenuous patient. A single hepatic vein can be sutured closed and, if necessary, the IVC can be significantly narrowed with sutures.

➤ Wisdom

Remember your liver principles of EIO; outflow control now means packing.

Do not let your hubris exceed that of your trauma colleague. If you cannot get the bleeding under control, repack, close and obtain an angiogram for arterial embolization. You can then get a good night's sleep. Large liver sutures may help with tamponade of hepatic venous bleeding. We use a 3.0 Prolene® suture on a large MH needle. Major liver resections do not end well in acidotic, coagulopathic patients. The only time to remove some liver is when the injury has done most of the work for you. Completing the 'resection' with a few strategic stapler applications will allow better exposure to the raw liver surface and then easy control with sutures.

You may be asked to attend the ritual pack removal a day or two later. Be sure to gather all the information you can about the initial operative findings. An updated CT may be very helpful in showing you the extent of the injury (i.e., is there involvement of the retrohepatic cava?). Put your retractor in place and ensure excellent exposure before starting to tease out the packs. If you get rebleeding do not think twice about repacking and trying again another day! It can be very helpful to cover the smashed liver with a non-sticky (i.e., plastic) bag during the initial packing procedure. The subsequent unpacking then avoids hemorrhage from the denuded liver upon removal. If plastic hasn't been placed, use lots of irrigation on the sponges, move slowly and don't forget your Aquamantys™ for help controlling parenchymal bleeding.

Injury to major Glissonian sheaths can result in postoperative bile leaks and sepsis in a large percentage of these patients. Drains and biliary stents will get you through. The body will manage large areas of devascularized liver if you have a little patience.

➢ Wisdom

The only liver to remove is when the injury has already done the resection.

The traumatised pancreas is unhappy and in a short period of time will get storming mad. You have a limited window to operate (24-48 hours). You should operate for ongoing bleeding/instability or suspected parenchymal transection. Complete exploration and drainage will be sufficient for most situations. A completely transected body or neck should prompt a distal pancreatectomy. If you suspect that the main pancreatic duct is torn, resection may avoid a reoperation; drainage still works. In a stable patient, intraoperative ultrasonography may help decision making. Dismiss the idea of doing an on-table pancreatogram. Trying to cannulate the pancreatic duct in a trauma situation is meddlesome. Similarly, an emergency ERCP is an unnecessary delay; suspected pancreatic injuries should be explored regardless of the result. The idea that you are going to successfully treat a damaged duct with an ERCP placed stent is a fantasy. Doing a pancreatojejunostomy to any part of a damaged or transected pancreas is to be avoided. You don't like sewing to a soft pancreas in the elective situation so why would you consider doing it in an emergency situation.

➤ Wisdom

A drain solves 90% of pancreatic trauma; only resect if you suspect a torn main duct.

Bleeding from the portal vein is an especially nasty situation. A rapid and extended Kocher maneuver will allow a hand to squeeze control this vein; this gives you time to work on the exposure. A detailed three-dimensional knowledge of this area will allow an HPB surgeon to gain this exposure without making things worse. The pancreatic neck may need to be divided to gain a proper view of bleeding. Ligation of the portal vein should be avoided, except as a last ditch attempt to save the patient. You are a vascular surgeon; sew the vein back together.

In the late 19th century, a young Alexis Carrel, eventual Nobel laureate and father of vascular surgery, criticized the surgeons that ligated the French President's portal vein after he was stabbed with a dagger. The President died; a blacklisted Carrel eventually emigrated to Canada.

➤ Wisdom

Divide the pancreatic neck to save a life.

If there is serious bleeding from the splenic vein or artery, you can typically get your hand around this structure. At this point of control, you can decide to repair or resect. As the pancreas is likely to be damaged, resection is often the best option.

Isolated duodenal injuries should be simply sutured. We use interrupted sutures so any failure is a leak and not a disruption. Major loss of duodenal tissue may require more creativity; remember that the duodenum is quite redundant and when mobilized can often be closed, transversely if necessary. We have never been great fans of pyloric exclusion. What exactly does it exclude? Considering the utility of an NG tube and the liters of biliary and pancreatic fluid that still flows through this area, the answer is — perhaps not much. Is it really worth doing a gastrojejunal anastomosis in a contaminated field?

 Wisdom

Pyloric exclusion is not an HPB operation.

Major disruption of the pancreaticoduodenal complex may require resection. This is not for patients in extremis. In these cases, suture control of bleeders and/or packing is indicated. If the patient survives the night, resection can be done the next day. Stable patients can undergo an expedited Whipple procedure; the reconstruction phase may have to be delayed, perhaps as much as 24 hours depending on the patient's condition.

 Wisdom

A trauma Whipple makes you a hero.

Gallbladder damage, in anything but an unstable patient, means cholecystectomy. Do not prosecute a cholecystectomy in a coagulopathic patient; just sew up the hole. Extrahepatic biliary injuries are mostly about controlling the surrounding vascular damage. Multiple large clamp applications to the porta hepatis can temporarily control bleeding in the porta hepatis. Only a very stable patient can undergo biliary reconstruction; otherwise, drainage is the right option.

One of the biggest dangers of inviting an HPB surgeon into a trauma OR is that he or she tries to do too much. Not being there from the beginning can result in a lack of understanding of the patient's instability: volume of blood loss and other injuries. It is important to sense the situation and have restraint. Let your trauma colleague teach you the art of bailing out with balloon tamponade or the placement of a temporary intravascular shunt.

Wisdoms

- *Remember your liver principles of EIO; outflow control now means packing.*

- *The only liver to remove is when the injury has already done the resection.*

- *A drain solves 90% of pancreatic trauma; only resect If you suspect a torn main duct.*

- *Divide the pancreatic neck to save a life.*

- *Pyloric exclusion is not an HPB operation.*

- *A trauma Whipple makes you a hero.*

Chapter 31

Critical care and the HPB surgeon

God will not look you over for medals, degrees or diplomas, but for scars.
Elbert Hubbard

The improved results of HPB surgery are, in part, the result of refinements in critical care. Extensive high-risk procedures on elderly patients can only be undertaken with the understanding of critical care back-up. Intensivists deserve our support and respect. Improvements in ventilator and ionotropic support combined with an improved understanding of the physiology of sepsis are responsible. Severely ill postoperative patients can be salvaged now when years ago they would have died. Months of support in harrowing circumstances can turn to a positive outcome.

An HPB surgeon who has a patient that has fallen into this abyss needs a strategy that allows both him and his patient to survive. Serious postoperative complications paint the surgeon with the brush of guilt and shame. A trip to the ICU exposes your leaks and bleeds to the world. Be humble. Be honest: full disclosure to the patient, family and intensivist. Stay involved with all three, especially when the process extends out over months. Having complications is part of the landscape and you will likely only be judged harshly if you abandon your patient. Reoperations while unpleasant are also part of the HPB world; avoidance will only make things worse. Only the operating surgeon has a true understanding of the intraabdominal process, what interventions are indicated and when. Drains and wound care remain the surgeon's responsibility. The patient and family still look to their surgeon for support and encouragement. While you cannot be there continuously, it is often useful to inform and involve a trusted colleague. You can get a break and deliver a fresh set of eyes on a difficult problem.

➢ Wisdom

Don't abandon your critical care HPB patient.

Operating on elderly people with deadly cancers can create ethical dilemmas when they enter the critical care unit. The poor oncological results with pancreatic cancer surgery may result in a postoperative complication being interpreted as a palliative situation. Consideration of care withdrawal may be premature. The HPB surgeon must guide this process and stand up for the patient in situations where things are not hopeless. Prolonging life can be as meaningful as saving life. A preoperative critical care consult and family discussions may avoid misunderstandings.

➢ Wisdom

A postoperative complication in an elderly cancer patient is not a palliative situation.

The other reason for an HPB surgeon to enter the critical care unit is severe acute pancreatitis. These desperately ill patients may require an operation. Decision making is hard, their course is complicated and their length of stay is prolonged. This often makes many of these unoperated patients undesirable. This is unfortunate as they are often young with a long future life at risk. Perhaps this is a good time to step up.

➤ Wisdom

Step up to the challenge of severe acute pancreatitis.

Wisdoms

- *Don't abandon your critical care HPB patient.*

- *A postoperative complication in an elderly cancer patient is not a palliative situation.*

- *Step up to the challenge of severe acute pancreatitis.*

Chapter 32

Pediatric HPB surgery

It's the little details that are vital.
Little things make big things happen.
John Wooden

Children are just small adults! Don't change your principles or good habits just because you are operating on tiny people. However, the key word here is small. You have to make an adjustment to your reality as distances are foreshortened. Your cognitive maps need to be miniaturized. Blood vessels and ducts that, in an adult, would be dismissed as insignificant, can be major structures. The splenic artery is the size of a pen nib in a 5-year-old. These differences are also variable with the different sizes of these youngsters. A mental adjustment to blood loss is also necessary. What seems like an acceptable amount of bleeding in a 5-year-old may actually be excessive because of their lower blood volume. An experienced pediatric anesthesiologist can help keep you and the patient on track.

➢ Wisdom

'Small' changes pediatric HPB operations.

Situational awareness is useful when interacting with your pediatric surgery colleagues. They come from a historical background where pediatric surgeons did all aspects of general surgery. The number of HPB surgical procedures needed for the pediatric population is small, so acquiring and maintaining expertise is difficult in all but the largest centers. A close collaboration between pediatric and HPB surgeons is a natural solution. If you are asked to help resect a liver or pancreas tumor in a pediatric patient, some upfront discussion on who is going to do which component of the operation is critical. Meeting with the patient and parents prior to the operation is also a good idea. Even if you are not on record as the primary operator, you still bear a heavy responsibility.

If you are operating in an unfamiliar hospital, be sure to have all your tools available. You should also be sure there is an appropriate retractor that fits the patient's size. A different retractor with smaller blades may have to be learned. Some change in technique may also be necessary as the size of the operative wound may not accommodate your mutton-sized hands. Operating in another institution also has the disadvantage of not having your colleagues to drop in and help in a sticky situation. An experienced HPB voice and hand is a comforting aid.

➢ Wisdom

The hands and voice of an experienced HPB colleague are irreplaceable.

For older and larger pediatric patients, considerations should be given to performing their surgery at your adult hospital. Consider transferring the patient to the children's facility postoperatively. This may be especially important if a laparoscopic approach is planned where tool substitution is unacceptable.

Wisdoms

- *'Small' changes pediatric HPB operations.*

- *The hands and voice of an experienced HPB colleague are irreplaceable.*

Epilogue

Parting thoughts

True merit, like a river, the deeper it is,
the less noise it makes.
Edward Wood, 1st Earl of Halifax

The writing of a book on 'wisdom' requires a certain amount of hubris. One might go so far as to say enough hubris to exclude any type of personal wisdom. Indeed, writing about wisdom does not mean one is wise, but rather that one has some insight into what it takes to become wise. Writing and doing are often not the same thing. Trying to acquire wisdom is a life-long struggle that is never really attained. If, at selected moments in your surgical career, you can look back and say "yes, at that moment I was wise", then you have succeeded. The 'unwise' moments need to be internalized without beating up the ego too much. We also have to recognize that some things are unknowable in advance. If we could remember to take time-outs in our regular lives, to actually ask ourselves if our present behavior is 'wise', perhaps we would all be better human beings.

 Wisdom

Use 'wisdom time-outs' outside the operating room.

Index

ablation therapy 132–3
abscess, liver 133
action bias 33, 180
adenoma, liver 134–5
adrenal glands 104, 290–1
alcohol abstinence 259
ALPPS procedures 94
ampulla of Vater 205, 247–9, 282, 284
anatomy 3, 41
    bile ducts 76, 78, 115–16, 148–9, 183, 220
    duodenum 221, 281–2
    gallbladder 165–9
    liver 13, 69–90, 105, 110, 115–16, 141
    pancreas 217–21
    porta hepatis 71, 73, 76, 77, 80, 148–51, 176
antibiotics 270
aortic clamping 101, 302
ascites 62, 226, 298
attention capacity 34
autoimmune pancreatitis 253–4
availability bias 33, 180

B-SAFE cholecystectomy landmarks 181–2
bad news 65–6
bail-out pathways 56

bariatric (gastric bypass) surgery 204
bile ducts
anatomy 76, 78, 115–16, 148–9, 183, 220
cholangiocarcinoma 139–40, 226, 293–4
dilated 158–9, 293–4
fistula 184–5, 211
Frey procedure 262, 263
injuries
due to electrocautery 119
during gallbladder removal 176–85
in the gallbladder plate 206
repair 191–9
to sectoral ducts 183–5, 195
traumatic 306
Mirizzi syndrome 207–9
not leaking 126
in the porta hepatis 151
hepaticojejunostomy 153–7, 191–2
recurrent pyogenic cholangitis 141–2
stents 139, 195, 252–3, 254
stones in 203–5
biliary cystadenoma 136–7
biopsies 92, 223–4
bleeding control 38–9, 47–8, 60–1
hepatic veins 114, 206–7
laparoscopies 125
liver 101–2, 114, 120–3, 138, 142, 301–3
pancreas 226–7, 239, 242, 246, 256, 272
portal vein 226–7, 304
splenectomy 290
trauma 301–6

Cantlie's line 73
caudate lobe 85–7, 120
cavernous malformations 160
central venous pressure (CVP) 101–2, 120, 301

checklists
    postoperative 126
    preoperative 23–4
children 311–12
cholangiocarcinoma 226, 293–4
    hilar 139–40
cholangiograms, intraoperative 205–6
cholangitis, recurrent 141–2
cholecystectomy 171, 185–6
    avoiding bile duct injuries 176–85
    in the cirrhotic patient 172, 297–8
    difficult/subtotal 187–90, 202
    gallbladder cancer 212–13
    laparoscopic ports 172–3, 201
    manipulation and navigation 173–6
    in morbidly obese patients 201
    open 151, 201–3
    in trauma patients 306
cholecystitis 168, 187–90, 202
    erosive 210–11
    Mirizzi syndrome 207–9
    pancreatic stenting 224–5
choledochal cysts 158–9
choledocholithiasis 203–5
cirrhotic patients 94, 123, 138, 172, 297–9
clips 38, 47
coeliac plexus blocks 251–2
cognitive biases 33–5, 75, 180–1
cognitive function (of patients) 52
cognitive heuristics 32–6, 44
cognitive maps 39, 43, 177–8
colon 285–6, 298
    mesentery 218
colorectal liver metastases 93, 94–5
communication
    bad news 65–6
    with other team members 9, 18–19, 22, 57
    with patients/families 28, 53, 57, 65–6, 192, 307

completing an operation 57, 126, 242
complications 35, 59–63
confirmation bias 33–4, 180–1
conflict (within teams) 19
consent 23
critical care 307–9
CT scans (computed tomography) 15, 48, 92, 223, 225
cystadenoma
     liver 135, 136–7
     pancreas 254
cystic artery 166
cystic duct 151, 166–8, 174, 207
cysts
     choledochal 158–9
     liver 135–6
     pancreas 254–6
     see also pseudocysts

dementia 52
diaphragm 119, 264
diathermy *see* electrocautery
dissection techniques 37–8
drains 57
     biliary 155, 192–3, 211
     pancreas 241, 242, 245, 265, 272, 274, 304
ducts of Luschka 206
duodenum
     anatomy 221, 281–2
     bile duct anastomosis 154
     diverticula 285
     gallstone in 210
     and pancreatic surgery 221, 229, 235–6, 248, 256
     resection 282–5
     trauma 305

echinococcosis 135–6
electrocautery 47–8, 119–20, 121, 122, 124, 240
     hook cautery 174, 183

embolization 138, 246
    portal vein 93, 94, 119
endoscopy
    debridement of pancreatic necrosum 273, 275–6
    ERCP 203–4, 256, 270
    ultrasound 223, 248
endostaplers 134, 239
equipment 24, 47–9
ERCP 203, 270
    complications 256
eschar plugs 122
exam table test 52

falciform ligament 69, 126
finishing an operation 57, 126, 242
flank approach (debridement of pancreatic necrosum) 274–5
flap incisions 96
focal nodular hyperplasia 134
Frey procedure 260–3
future liver remnant (FLR) 93–4

gallbladder 164
    anatomy 165–9
    cancer 212–13
    cholangiography, intraoperative 205–6
    cholecystectomy see cholecystectomy
    cholecystitis 168, 187–90, 202
        erosive 210–11
        pancreatic stenting 224–5
    gallstone removal 188–90, 202, 203–5
    Mirizzi syndrome 207–9
    sump syndrome 211
    varices 168, 297–8
    wisdoms 169, 185–6, 190, 199, 213–14
gallbladder plate 76, 165
    injuries 206–7
gastric conditions/surgery see stomach

gastrocolic trunk 219, 228
gastroduodenal artery (GDA) 152, 220, 229–30, 261
gastroepiploic artery 238, 287
Glissonian sheaths 78–9, 82, 111–12, 253, 303
Glisson's capsule 69, 83
go/no go decision 51–4

'hanging liver' technique 119
haptics 33
Hartmann's pouch 168
heart failure 142
hemangioma, liver 133–4, 142
hemihepatectomy 95, 109–19, 141
hemostasis see bleeding control
hepatic arteries
    anatomy 76, 78, 111, 150, 151, 152
    in cholecystectomy 179
    injured 191, 196
    in pancreatic surgery 229–30, 246, 253
hepatic conditions/surgery see liver
hepatic duct 148–9, 151, 178, 183, 193, 197
hepatic veins
    anatomy 80, 87–8
    bleeding control 101, 114, 125, 206
    dissection 105–7
    in liver resections 117–18
    trauma 302
hepaticojejunostomy 153–7, 191–2
hepatobiliary triangle 166, 173–5
hepatocellular cancer (HCC) 94, 131, 132, 138
hepatoduodenal ligament see porta hepatis
hernias 298
heuristics 31–40, 44
hilar plate 76, 77–8, 110, 148
    injuries 119–20, 195–7
hilum (liver) 81, 110
    cholangiocarcinoma 139–40

history of HPB surgery 1–2, 13–15
hook cautery 174, 183
hydatid cysts 135–6

imaging 15, 48
    cholangiography 205–6
    intraoperative 98, 108, 205–6
    liver 91–2, 98, 108, 134
    pancreas 223, 225, 253, 254, 255
incisions
    for cholecystectomy 203
    duodenal 282
    for liver surgery 95–7
    for pancreatic surgery 227–8, 236
inferior vena cava (IVC)
    anatomy 88–9
    clamping 101–2
    dissection 104–6
    trauma 302
inferior vena cava ligament 88, 104
interpersonal skills 9, 18–19, 22–3, 57
intraductal papillary mucinous neoplasms (IPMN) 254–5, 294–5
'invisible vein flaps' 231–2
IVC *see* inferior vena cava

kidneys 291
Kocher maneuver 228, 248

laparoscopy 14, 39–40, 48–50
    cholecystectomy 171–86, 201
    liver ablation 132–3
    liver resection 123–6
    pancreatic operations 226, 240–1, 250
    port placement 124, 172–3, 201
leadership 22–3
learning 41–6, 197
left triangular/coronary ligament 70

ligament of Treitz 221
lighting 37
liver 1–2, 68
    ablation therapy 132–3
    abscess 133
    anatomy 13, 69–90, 105, 110, 115–16, 141
    benign tumors 134–5
    bleeding control 101–2, 114, 120–3, 138, 142, 301–3
    caudate resection 120
    central resection 119–20
    cirrhotic patients 94, 123, 138, 172, 297–9
    congenital anomalies 294
    cystadenoma 135, 136–7
    cysts 135–6
    dissection of IVC and hepatic veins 104–7
    EIO (exposure, inflow control, outflow control) 99–102, 110–12, 116, 120–3, 124–5, 301
    failure 98, 131–2
    and heart failure 142
    hemangioma 133–4, 142
    hemihepatectomy 109–10, 119
        plus colon resection 95
        left 116–18
        right 110–16, 119
    hilar cholangiocarcinoma 139–40
    imaging 91–2, 134
        intraoperative 98, 108
    incisions 95–7
    laparoscopy 123–6, 132–3
    mobilization 70, 71–2, 102–4
    neuroendocrine metastases 138
    parenchymal dissection 120–3
    porta hepatis *see* porta hepatis
    portosystemic shunts 142–3
    postoperative checks 126
    preoperative planning 91–5
    recurrent pyogenic cholangitis 141–2

repeat hepatectomy 141
retractors 97, 99
segmental resection 108–9, 123, 124
transplantation 131, 143
trauma 301–3
wisdoms 90, 127–9, 144
lymph nodes
    cystic duct 166, 176
    porta hepatis 152

mesohepatectomy 119–20
microwave ablation 132
mindfulness 25
minimally invasive surgery *see* laparoscopy
Mirizzi syndrome 207–9
mistakes 10, 35, 42
    documentation 192
motor heuristics 36–40
MRI (magnetic resonance imaging) 48, 92, 134, 223
multidisciplinary teams 17–20, 21–3, 27–8

necrotizing pancreatitis 256, 267–77, 308–9
neuroendocrine liver metastases 138
night staff 62

obesity 56–7, 201
obliquity of the liver 73–5
operating room environment 21–5
operating tables 37, 274
outcome reviews 27–8

pain 133–4
    in pancreatitis 251–2, 259
pancreas 1–2, 216
    acute (necrotizing) pancreatitis 256, 267–77, 308–9
    ampullary resection 247–9
    anatomy 217–21

autoimmune pancreatitis 253–4
bleeding control 226–7, 239, 242, 246, 256, 272
borderline resectable tumors 247
central pancreas surgery 241
chronic pancreatitis 259–66, 294
congenital anomalies 295
cysts 254–6
distal pancreatectomy (left pancreas) 236–41, 264, 288
drains 241, 242, 245, 265, 272, 274, 304
enucleation of tumors 250
ERCP complications 256
fistulas 265, 272, 275
Frey procedure 260–3
imaging 223, 225, 253, 254, 255
incisions 227–8, 236
IPMN 254–5, 294–5
laparoscopy 226, 240–1, 250
leaks 61, 235, 245–7, 250
palliation 250–3, 308
preoperative procedures 223–6
pseudocysts 265, 267–8, 276
trauma 303–4
Whipple procedure 14, 228–36, 264–5, 284, 287, 305
wisdoms 221, 242–3, 257, 266, 277
pancreatic duct 220, 250
dilated 294–5
Frey procedure 260
pancreatic divisum 295
pancreaticobiliary maljunction 158
stenting 224–5
trauma 303
pancreaticoduodenectomy *see* Whipple procedure
parabiliary venous system 151
patients
communication with 28, 53, 57, 65–6, 192, 307
position on table 99, 124
who to operate on 51–4

pediatric surgery 311–12
peritoneum 69–70
pinch burning 38
plates of the liver 76
    gallbladder plate 76, 165, 206–7
    hilar plate 76, 77–8, 110, 119–20, 148, 195–7
    plate of Arantius 76
    umbilical plate 76, 84
pleural cavity, fistula from pancreas 265
polycystic liver disease 134
porta hepatis (hepatoduodenal ligament) 146–61
    anatomy 71, 73, 76, 77, 80, 148–51, 176
    cavernous malformations 160
    choledochal cysts 158–9
    hepaticojejunostomy 153–7, 191–2
    operating on 151–2
    redo hepatectomy 141
portal hypertension 225, 290
portal vein
    anatomy 76, 84, 150, 218
    bleeding control 226–7, 304
    borderline resectable pancreatic tumors 247
    cavernous malformations 160
    embolization 93, 94, 119
    injuries 191, 253, 304
    reconstruction 139–40
    trauma 305
    in the Whipple procedure 228–9, 231, 236
portosystemic shunts 142–3
positioning
    patients 99, 124
    surgeons 36, 37
postoperative care 59–63
    bile duct injuries 192, 198
    critical care 307–9
    liver surgery 126
    pancreatic surgery 245–7

preoperative period
    liver surgery 91–5
    pancreatic surgery 223–6
    patient assessment 51–4
    surgical checklists 23–4
primacy bias (first impressions) 33
Pringle maneuver 100, 125
pseudocysts, pancreatic 265, 267–8, 276
PVE (portal vein embolization) 93, 94, 119
pyloric exclusion 305

quality of care 27–9

radiofrequency ablation 132–3
recurrent pyogenic cholangitis 141–2
retractors 97, 99, 203, 312
robotics 49
rule of Ts 246
Rumel tourniquets 100, 121

second opinions 51, 53, 197–8, 308
sectoral/segmental liver anatomy 80–2
sepsis 61, 269
skill development 41–6, 197
SMA (superior mesenteric artery) 220, 232–3
smoking cessation 259
SMV (superior mesenteric vein) 218, 220, 228
sphincter of Oddi 256, 295
Spiegel lobe 85, 120
splanchnic veins 218–19
spleen 238, 240, 264, 287–90
splenic artery 220, 239, 240, 290, 304–5
splenic vein 219, 236, 237, 240, 290, 304–5
stapling 39, 239, 241
stents
    biliary 139, 195, 252–3, 254
    pancreatic 224–5

stereotactic body radiotherapy 132
stomach
    anatomy 286–7
    bypass (bariatric) surgery 204
    outlet obstruction 62–3, 251, 276
    transgastric debridement of pancreatic necrosum 272–4
    varices 238, 290
    in the Whipple procedure 230–1, 287
suckers 174, 190
sump syndrome 211
superior mesenteric artery (SMA) 220, 232–3
superior mesenteric vein (SMV) 218, 220, 228
surgical errors (mistakes) 10, 35, 42
    documentation 192
Surgical Safety Checklist 23–4
surgical techniques 37–9
suturing 39, 125–6, 233–4

T-tubes 205
teamwork 17–20, 21–3, 27–8
time-outs 34, 35, 56, 57, 60, 182, 313
tissue assessment 55–6
total vascular exclusion (TVE) 101
touch, sense of 33
training 41–6, 197
transduodenal sphincteroplasty 205
transplantation, liver 131, 143
trauma surgery 301–6

ultrasound (US)
    ampulla 223, 248
    liver (intraoperative) 98, 108
umbilical fossa 83–5
umbilical plate 76, 84

varices 142, 168, 172, 238, 290, 297–8

vascular anatomy
    bile duct 148
    gallbladder 166
    liver 80, 87–9, 105, 110
        porta hepatis 150–1
    pancreas 218–19
    spleen 287–8
    stomach 286–7
    see also individual vessels

Warshaw procedure 287
Whipple procedure 14, 228–36, 284, 287
    in chronic pancreatitis 264–5
    in trauma 305
wisdom 7–12, 313